Applying Systems Thinking to Regenerative Medicine

PROCEEDINGS OF A WORKSHOP

Siobhan Addie, Meredith Hackmann, Lydia Teferra, Anna Nicholson, and Sarah H. Beachy, *Rapporteurs*

Forum on Regenerative Medicine

Board on Health Sciences Policy

Health and Medicine Division

The National Academies of
SCIENCES • ENGINEERING • MEDICINE

THE NATIONAL ACADEMIES PRESS
Washington, DC
www.nap.edu

THE NATIONAL ACADEMIES PRESS   500 Fifth Street, NW   Washington, DC 20001

This activity was supported by contracts between the National Academy of Sciences and Advanced Regenerative Manufacturing Institute; Akron Biotech; Alliance for Regenerative Medicine; American Society of Gene & Cell Therapy; Burroughs Wellcome Fund (Grant No. 1021433); California Institute for Regenerative Medicine; Centre for Commercialization of Regenerative Medicine; Department of Veterans Affairs (Contract No. VA26816C0051P00004); Food and Drug Administration: Office of the Commissioner and Center for Biologics Evaluation and Research (Grant No. 1R13FD006614-02); International Society for Cellular Therapy; International Society for Stem Cell Research; Johnson & Johnson; The Michael J. Fox Foundation for Parkinson's Research; National Institute of Standards and Technology; National Institutes of Health (Contract No. HHSN263201800029I; Order No. 75N98019F00847): National Center for Advancing Translational Sciences; National Eye Institute; National Heart, Lung, and Blood Institute; National Institute of Biomedical Imaging and Bioengineering; National Institute of Dental and Craniofacial Research; National Institute of Diabetes and Digestive and Kidney Diseases; National Institute of Neurological Disorders and Stroke; National Institute on Aging; The New York Stem Cell Foundation; and Sanofi (Contract No. 55630791). Any opinions, findings, conclusions, or recommendations expressed in this publication do not necessarily reflect the views of any organization or agency that provided support for the project.

International Standard Book Number-13: 978-0-309-15182-5
International Standard Book Number-10: 0-309-15182-1
Digital Object Identifier: https://doi.org/10.17226/26025

Additional copies of this publication are available from the National Academies Press, 500 Fifth Street, NW, Keck 360, Washington, DC 20001; (800) 624-6242 or (202) 334-3313; http://www.nap.edu.

Copyright 2021 by the National Academy of Sciences. All rights reserved.

Printed in the United States of America

Suggested citation: National Academies of Sciences, Engineering, and Medicine. 2021. *Applying systems thinking to regenerative medicine: Proceedings of a workshop.* Washington, DC: The National Academies Press. https://doi.org/10.17226/26025.

The National Academies of
SCIENCES · ENGINEERING · MEDICINE

The **National Academy of Sciences** was established in 1863 by an Act of Congress, signed by President Lincoln, as a private, nongovernmental institution to advise the nation on issues related to science and technology. Members are elected by their peers for outstanding contributions to research. Dr. Marcia McNutt is president.

The **National Academy of Engineering** was established in 1964 under the charter of the National Academy of Sciences to bring the practices of engineering to advising the nation. Members are elected by their peers for extraordinary contributions to engineering. Dr. John L. Anderson is president.

The **National Academy of Medicine** (formerly the Institute of Medicine) was established in 1970 under the charter of the National Academy of Sciences to advise the nation on medical and health issues. Members are elected by their peers for distinguished contributions to medicine and health. Dr. Victor J. Dzau is president.

The three Academies work together as the **National Academies of Sciences, Engineering, and Medicine** to provide independent, objective analysis and advice to the nation and conduct other activities to solve complex problems and inform public policy decisions. The National Academies also encourage education and research, recognize outstanding contributions to knowledge, and increase public understanding in matters of science, engineering, and medicine.

Learn more about the National Academies of Sciences, Engineering, and Medicine at www.nationalacademies.org.

The National Academies of
SCIENCES • ENGINEERING • MEDICINE

Consensus Study Reports published by the National Academies of Sciences, Engineering, and Medicine document the evidence-based consensus on the study's statement of task by an authoring committee of experts. Reports typically include findings, conclusions, and recommendations based on information gathered by the committee and the committee's deliberations. Each report has been subjected to a rigorous and independent peer-review process and it represents the position of the National Academies on the statement of task.

Proceedings published by the National Academies of Sciences, Engineering, and Medicine chronicle the presentations and discussions at a workshop, symposium, or other event convened by the National Academies. The statements and opinions contained in proceedings are those of the participants and are not endorsed by other participants, the planning committee, or the National Academies.

For information about other products and activities of the National Academies, please visit www.nationalacademies.org/about/whatwedo.

PLANNING COMMITTEE ON APPLYING SYSTEMS THINKING TO REGENERATIVE MEDICINE[1]

ANNE PLANT (*Co-Chair*), Fellow, National Institute of Standards and Technology
KRISHNENDU ROY (*Co-Chair*), Robert A. Milton Chair and Professor; Technical Lead, National Cell Manufacturing Consortium, Georgia Institute of Technology
TOM BOLLENBACH, Chief Technology Officer, Advanced Regenerative Manufacturing Institute
JAMIE HAMILTON, (former) Senior Associate Director, Research Programs, The Michael J. Fox Foundation for Parkinson's Research
DEBORAH HOSHIZAKI, Program Director, Division of Kidney, Urologic, and Hematologic Diseases, National Institute of Diabetes and Digestive and Kidney Diseases, National Institutes of Health
SADIK KASSIM, Chief Technology Officer, Vor Biopharma
MALCOM MOOS, Medical Officer and Senior Investigator, Center for Biologics Evaluation and Research, Food and Drug Administration
PHIL VANEK, Partner, Gamma Biosciences
CLAUDIA ZYLBERBERG, Chief Executive Officer, Akron Biotech

Forum on Regenerative Medicine Staff

SARAH H. BEACHY, Senior Program Officer and Forum Director
SIOBHAN ADDIE, Program Officer
MEREDITH HACKMANN, Associate Program Officer
LYDIA TEFERRA, Research Assistant

Board on Health Sciences Policy Staff

BRIDGET BOREL, Program Coordinator
ANDREW M. POPE, Senior Board Director

---

[1] The National Academies of Sciences, Engineering, and Medicine's planning committees are solely responsible for organizing the workshop, identifying topics, and choosing speakers. The responsibility for the published Proceedings of a Workshop rests with the workshop rapporteurs and the institution.

FORUM ON REGENERATIVE MEDICINE[1]

TIM COETZEE (*Co-Chair*), Chief Advocacy, Services, and Science Officer, National Multiple Sclerosis Society
KATHERINE TSOKAS (*Co-Chair*), Vice President, Regulatory, Quality, Risk Management and Drug Safety, Janssen Inc. Canada
SANGEETA BHATIA, John J. and Dorothy Wilson Professor, Institute for Medical Engineering and Science, Electrical Engineering and Computer Science, Massachusetts Institute of Technology
PHILIP JOHN BROOKS, Program Director, Office of Rare Disease Research, National Center for Advancing Translational Sciences, National Institutes of Health
GEORGE Q. DALEY, Director, Stem Cell Transplantation Program, Boston Children's Hospital and Dana-Farber Cancer Institute; Dean, Harvard Medical School
BRIAN FISKE, Senior Vice President, Research Programs, The Michael J. Fox Foundation for Parkinson's Research
LAWRENCE GOLDSTEIN, Distinguished Professor, Department of Cellular and Molecular Medicine, Department of Neurosciences; Director, University of California, San Diego, Stem Cell Program; Scientific Director, Sanford Consortium for Regenerative Medicine; Director, Sanford Stem Cell Clinical Center, University of California, San Diego, School of Medicine
CANDACE KERR, Program Officer, Stem Cell Program, Aging Physiology Branch Division of Aging Biology, National Institute on Aging, National Institutes of Health
ROBERT S. LANGER, David H. Koch Institute Professor, Massachusetts Institute of Technology
CATO T. LAURENCIN, University Professor, Albert and Wilda Van Dusen Distinguished Professor of Orthopaedic Surgery, Professor of Chemical, Materials Science, and Biomedical Engineering; Director, The Raymond and Beverly Sackler Center for Biomedical, Biological, Physical, and Engineering Sciences; Chief Executive Officer, Connecticut Convergence Institute for Translation in Regenerative Engineering, University of Connecticut
TERRY MAGNUSON, Sarah Graham Kenan Professor, Vice Chancellor for Research, University of North Carolina at Chapel Hill
MICHAEL MAY, President and Chief Executive Officer, Centre for Commercialization of Regenerative Medicine

---

[1]The National Academies of Sciences, Engineering, and Medicine's forums and roundtables do not issue, review, or approve individual documents. The responsibility for the published Proceedings of a Workshop rests with the workshop rapporteurs and the institution.

RICHARD McFARLAND, Chief Regulatory Officer, Advanced Regenerative Manufacturing Institute
JACK MOSHER, Senior Manager, Scientific Affairs, International Society for Stem Cell Research
DAVID OWENS, Acting Deputy Director, Division of Extramural Research, National Institute of Neurological Disorders and Stroke, National Institutes of Health
AMY PATTERSON, Chief Science Advisor and Director of Scientific Research Programs, National Heart, Lung, and Blood Institute, National Institutes of Health
DUANQING PEI, Director General, Guangzhou Institutes of Biomedicine and Health, Chinese Academy of Sciences
ANNE PLANT, Chief of the Biosystems and Biomaterials Division, National Institute of Standards and Technology
KIMBERLEE POTTER, Scientific Program Manager, Biomedical Laboratory R&D Service, Office of Research and Development, Department of Veterans Affairs
DAVID RAMPULLA, Director, Division of Discovery Science and Technology (Bioengineering), Delivery Systems and Devices for Drugs and Biologics Synthetic Biological Systems, National Institute of Biomedical Imaging and Bioengineering, National Institutes of Health
DEREK ROBERTSON, Co-Founder and President, Maryland Sickle Cell Disease Association
KELLY ROSE, Program Officer, Burroughs Wellcome Fund
KRISHNENDU ROY, Robert A. Milton Chair and Professor in Biomedical Engineering; Technical Lead, National Cell Manufacturing Consortium; Director, Marcus Center for Therapeutic Cell Characterization and Manufacturing, Georgia Institute of Technology
KRISHANU SAHA, Associate Professor and Retina Research Foundation Kathryn and Latimer Murfee Chair, Department of Biomedical Engineering, University of Wisconsin–Madison
RACHEL SALZMAN, Society Officer, American Society of Gene & Cell Therapy
IVONNE SCHULMAN, Program Director, National Institute of Diabetes and Digestive and Kidney Diseases, National Institutes of Health
JAY P. SIEGEL, (retired) Chief Biotechnology Officer and Head, Scientific Strategy and Policy, Johnson & Johnson
LANA SKIRBOLL, Vice President, Science Policy, Sanofi
SUSAN L. SOLOMAN, Founder and Chief Executive Officer, The New York Stem Cell Foundation
MARTHA SOMERMAN, (former) Director, National Institute of Dental and Craniofacial Research, National Institutes of Health

MICHAEL STEINMETZ, Director, Division of Extramural Science Programs, National Eye Institute, National Institutes of Health
SOHEL TALIB, Associate Director of Therapeutics and Industry Alliance, California Institute for Regenerative Medicine
DANIEL WEISS, Chief Scientific Officer, International Society for Cellular Therapy
MICHAEL WERNER, Co-Founder and Senior Policy Counsel, Alliance for Regenerative Medicine
CELIA WITTEN, Deputy Director, Center for Biologics Evaluation and Research, Food and Drug Administration
CLAUDIA ZYLBERBERG, Founder and Chief Executive Officer, Akron Biotech

Forum on Regenerative Medicine Staff

SARAH H. BEACHY, Senior Program Officer and Forum Director
SIOBHAN ADDIE, Program Officer
MEREDITH HACKMANN, Associate Program Officer
LYDIA TEFERRA, Research Assistant

Board on Health Sciences Policy Staff

BRIDGET BOREL, Program Coordinator
ANDREW M. POPE, Senior Board Director

Reviewers

This Proceedings of a Workshop was reviewed in draft form by individuals chosen for their diverse perspectives and technical expertise. The purpose of this independent review is to provide candid and critical comments that will assist the National Academies of Sciences, Engineering, and Medicine in making each published proceedings as sound as possible and to ensure that it meets the institutional standards for quality, objectivity, evidence, and responsiveness to the charge. The review comments and draft manuscript remain confidential to protect the integrity of the process.

We thank the following individuals for their review of this proceedings:

MARTHA LUNDBERG, National Heart, Lung, and Blood Institute
RYAN MURPHY, National Academies of Sciences, Engineering, and Medicine
GUNARETNAM RAJAGOPAL, Johnson & Johnson

Although the reviewers listed above provided many constructive comments and suggestions, they were not asked to endorse the content of the proceedings nor did they see the final draft before its release. The review of this proceedings was overseen by **LINDA DEGUTIS,** Henry M. Jackson Foundation for the Advancement of Military Medicine. She was responsible for making certain that an independent examination of this proceedings was carried out in accordance with standards of the National Academies and that all review comments were carefully considered. Responsibility for the final content rests entirely with the rapporteurs and the National Academies.

Acknowledgments

The support of the sponsors of the Forum on Regenerative Medicine was crucial to the planning and conduct of the workshop Applying Systems Thinking to Regenerative Medicine and for the development of this Proceedings of a Workshop. Federal sponsors were the Department of Veterans Affairs; Food and Drug Administration: Office of the Commissioner and Center for Biologics Evaluation and Research; National Institute of Standards and Technology; and National Institutes of Health: National Center for Advancing Translational Sciences; National Eye Institute; National Heart, Lung, and Blood Institute; National Institute of Biomedical Imaging and Bioengineering; National Institute of Dental and Craniofacial Research; National Institute of Diabetes and Digestive and Kidney Diseases; National Institute of Neurological Disorders and Stroke; and National Institute on Aging. Nonfederal sponsorship was provided by Advanced Regenerative Manufacturing Institute; Akron Biotech; Alliance for Regenerative Medicine; American Society of Gene & Cell Therapy; Burroughs Wellcome Fund; California Institute for Regenerative Medicine; Centre for Commercialization of Regenerative Medicine; International Society for Cellular Therapy; International Society for Stem Cell Research; Johnson & Johnson; The Michael J. Fox Foundation for Parkinson's Research; The New York Stem Cell Foundation; and Sanofi.

The Forum on Regenerative Medicine wishes to express gratitude to the expert speakers who explored how cross-disciplinary systems thinking approaches can support the development of safe and effective regenerative medicine therapies. The forum also wishes to thank the members of the planning committee for their work in developing an excellent workshop agenda. The project director would like to thank the project staff who worked diligently to develop both the workshop and the resulting Proceedings of a Workshop.

Contents

ACRONYMS AND ABBREVIATIONS   xix

1   INTRODUCTION   1
Organization of the Proceedings, 7

2   INTRODUCTION TO SYSTEMS THINKING CONCEPTS   9
An Introduction to Systems Thinking, 10
Applying Systems Thinking to the Development of
    Regenerative Medicines, 16
Systems Dynamics of Cell-State Transitions: Relevance
    for Regenerative Medicine, 20
Discussion, 24

3   EXPLORING THE CHALLENGES OF CRITICAL
QUALITY ATTRIBUTES: THE ROLE OF
SYSTEMS THINKING   29
Systems Thinking and the Regulation of Regenerative
    Medicine Products, 31
Using Systems Thinking Approaches for Cell Therapy
    Product Development, 37
Discussion, 41

4	CHALLENGES ASSOCIATED WITH DATA COLLECTION, AGGREGATION, AND SHARING	47

Toward Open Science in Omics Analysis and
  Disease Modeling, 48
Using Big Data for Clinical Stratification of Patients, 53
Discussion, 58

5	CHALLENGES AND OPPORTUNITIES ASSOCIATED WITH SYSTEMS-LEVEL ANALYSIS AND MODELING	65

Developing Algorithms for Single-Cell Genomics, 66
Modeling Dynamic Data to Identify a Latent Space, 70
Adopting Metabolic Modeling Tools in Biopharmaceutical
  Drug Development, 74
Discussion, 78

6	ADDRESSING REGENERATIVE MEDICINE MANUFACTURING AND SUPPLY CHAIN CHALLENGES WITH SYSTEMS-LEVEL APPROACHES	85

Artificial Intelligence in Cell and Gene Therapies, 86
Modeling the Manufacturing Process in Regenerative Medicine, 91
Novel Supply Chain and Cost Modeling for Cell Therapies, 98
Discussion, 103

7	EXPLORING ISSUES OF WORKFORCE DEVELOPMENT RELATED TO SYSTEMS THINKING	109

Education and Workforce Development to Advance
  Systems Thinking, 110
Reflections on the Workshop, 116
Final Words on Models and Data, 118

REFERENCES   121

APPENDIXES
A WORKSHOP AGENDA   127
B SPEAKER BIOGRAPHICAL SKETCHES   137
C STATEMENT OF TASK   149

Boxes, Figures, and Tables

BOXES

1-1 Workshop Statement of Task, 3

6-1 Grand Challenges in Cell Manufacturing, 92
6-2 Questions to Consider in Determining Analysis Objectives, 97

FIGURES

1-1 Cell therapy: interaction of multi-scale dynamic complex systems, 5
1-2 A systems approach to inform the regenerative medicine field, 6

2-1 Fruit fly early development: from maternal inputs to larva, 12

3-1 Process of cell therapy development as a system, 39

6-1 Complexity of regenerative medicine supply chain ecosystem, 99

TABLES

4-1 Use Cases for Real-World Data, 59

6-1 Factors Influencing Each Stage in the Development of Autologous Cell Therapies, 90

Acronyms and Abbreviations

ACO	accountable care organization
AD	Alzheimer's disease
AI	artificial intelligence
AMP AD	Accelerating Medicines Partnership Alzheimer's Disease
APC	antigen-presenting cells
AUC	area under the curve
CAR	chimeric antigen receptor
CMaT	Cell Manufacturing Technologies
CoGAPS	Coordinated Gene Activity in Pattern Sets
CPP	critical process parameter
CQA	critical quality attribute
CRS	cytokine release syndrome
DREAM	Dialogue on Reverse Engineering Assessment and Methods
EHR	electronic health record
ERC	engineering research center
FDA	Food and Drug Administration
FHIR	Fast Healthcare Interoperability Resources
GMP	good manufacturing practice

HIPAA	Health Insurance Portability and Accountability Act
iPS	induced pluripotent stem
MOA	mechanism of action
NCI	National Cancer Institute
NIH	National Institutes of Health
NIIMBL	National Institute for Innovation in Manufacturing Biopharmaceuticals
NIST	National Institute of Standards and Technology
NLP	natural language processing
NMR	nuclear magnetic resonance
NSF	National Science Foundation
OMOP	Observational Medical Outcomes Partnership
PCORI	Patient-Centered Outcomes Research Institute
PD	Parkinson's disease
QC	quality control
RM	regenerative medicine
SBIR	Small Business Innovation Research
STTR	Small Business Technology Transfer
TCR	T cell receptor
UCH	University of California Health (system)
UMAP	Uniform Manifold Approximation and Projection

1

Introduction[1]

Regenerative medicine products, which are intended to repair or replace damaged cells or tissues in the body, include a range of therapeutic approaches such as cell- and gene-based therapies, engineered tissues, and non-biologic constructs. It is often challenging to properly characterize these products for a number of reasons. The mechanisms of action of these products (i.e., the biochemistry that results in their therapeutic result) is incompletely understood, the complexity of intracellular and biochemical networks is confounding, and complicated patient responses to therapies involve variable interactions within patients' cellular and physiological microenvironments. As a result, there is often not a definitive correlation between what is measured and the clinical outcome for these complex products. Additional complexity is introduced by the manufacturing process and by the difficulty in predicting the biological effect of these processes. It is important to understand which measurements accurately and reliably characterize products in a way that is predictive of their clinical efficacy and safety for patients.

The quality attributes of regenerative medicine products was a topic of discussion at a previous public workshop of the Forum on Regenerative

---

[1] The planning committee's role was limited to planning the workshop, and the Proceedings of a Workshop was prepared by the workshop rapporteurs as a factual summary of what occurred at the workshop. Statements, recommendations, and opinions expressed are those of individual presenters and participants, and are not necessarily endorsed or verified by the National Academies of Sciences, Engineering, and Medicine, and they should not be construed as reflecting any group consensus.

Medicine (NASEM, 2017). These attributes can include identity, quantity, purity, sterility, viability, and potency, and are measured and validated as part of regulatory submissions. Reliable characterization of regenerative medicine products is required to ensure quality, safety, and efficacy; these characteristics are identified as the products' critical quality attributes (CQAs) (Burke and Zylberberg, 2019). However, to the extent that each product has unique features, it is likely that each product requires unique assays for characterization. The exact mechanisms of action for many regenerative medicine products are not well understood, making it difficult to determine which factors or analytes need to be measured to assess biological activity or identity (Tsokas et al., 2019). An additional challenge in defining CQAs is that in vitro metrics are not always predictive of in vivo activity. One approach to characterization might be to measure numerous assay endpoints, but this is a potentially expensive and unsustainable approach. Furthermore, collecting large amounts of data in the absence of an appropriate theoretical construct or clear understanding of mechanism of action may not elucidate the most important characteristics of a given product or system that provide the predictive information needed by researchers, manufacturers, and regulators.

A systems-focused approach is intended to better define the mechanistic parameters involved in the biological outcome and allows for the collection and use of more relevant data by recognizing those analytes that are most indicative of providing the most important predictive and actionable information about a product. Systems thinking[2] involves the consideration of data acquisition, data analysis, and theoretical frameworks in order to develop a predictive understanding of complex systems. It is a multidisciplinary effort and can incorporate tools and knowledge from the fields of data science, biology, engineering, manufacturing, regulatory science, and clinical research and therefore requires the use of disparate data sources. Systems thinking for regenerative medicine might involve consideration of the characteristics of starting materials, ancillary materials, manufacturing processes, and patient characteristics in models that consider the physical factors that control the regulatory pathways associated with a given therapeutic outcome.

---

[2] The term "systems thinking" does not currently have a widely accepted definition. However, the concept of systems thinking is closely associated with "developing coherent understanding of complex biological processes and phenomena from the molecular level to the level of ecosystems" (Verhoeff et al., 2018). According to one proposed definition, "Systems thinking is a set of synergistic analytic skills used to improve the capability of identifying and understanding systems, predicting their behaviors, and devising modifications to them in order to produce desired effects. These skills work together as a system" (Arnold and Wade, 2015, p. 675). See Chapter 2 for additional discussion of the definition of systems thinking by the workshop speakers.

Given these considerations, the Forum on Regenerative Medicine convened experts across disciplines for a 2-day virtual public workshop to explore systems thinking approaches and how they may be applied to support the identification of relevant quality attributes that can help in the optimization of manufacturing and streamline regulatory processes for regenerative medicine. The Statement of Task for the workshop can be found in Box 1-1. A broad array of stakeholders participated in the workshop, including data scientists, physical scientists, industry researchers, regulatory officials, clinicians, and patient representatives.

In opening the workshop, the planning committee members Anne Plant, a National Institutes of Standards and Technology (NIST) fellow and the former chief of the Biosystems and Biomaterials Division at NIST, and Krishnendu Roy, the Robert A. Milton Chair Professor, the director of the National Science Foundation's Engineering Research Center for Cell Manufacturing Technologies, and the director of the Marcus Center for Therapeutic Cell Characterization and Manufacturing at the Wallace H. Coulter Department of Biomedical Engineering at the Georgia Institute of Technology and Emory University, described the workshop's motivation and focus. The primary objective in convening the workshop, Plant said, was to explore the challenges that could lead the field to identifying meaningful predictive CQAs (e.g., determining what should be measured about a product to best characterize it and predict how well the product will

---

BOX 1-1
Workshop Statement of Task

The current approach to characterizing the quality of a regenerative medicine product and the manufacturing process often involves measuring as many endpoints as possible, but this approach has proved to be inadequate and unsustainable. To explore how cross-disciplinary systems thinking approaches can support the identification of relevant quality attributes and streamline manufacturing and regulatory processes of regenerative medicine products, a planning committee of the National Academies of Sciences, Engineering, and Medicine will hold a public workshop. Speakers at the workshop may be asked to discuss new advances in data acquisition, data analysis and theoretical frameworks, and how systems approaches can be applied to the development of regenerative medicine products that can address the unmet needs of patients. Discussions may explore how systems thinking is currently being applied in clinical and manufacturing settings. The planning committee will develop the workshop agenda, select and invite speakers and discussants, and may moderate the discussions. A proceedings of the workshop will be prepared by a designated rapporteur in accordance with institutional guidelines.

work in a patient). This is a challenging task from the perspectives of both regulators and practitioners. Given the complexity of cell-based therapies, no single measure will suffice, yet it is difficult to determine which combination of measures will be predictive of the efficacy and safety of a product. Even for successful therapies with known benefit, measurements have not yet been sufficiently correlated with patients' clinical outcomes (Xue et al., 2017). New approaches and tools are needed to better understand the functional characteristics of the types of products emerging in the field of regenerative medicine, she said.

Another objective of the workshop was to explore challenges related to the increasing volumes of data that are now being collected, primarily through omics-type technologies. These data need to be parsed, analyzed, and integrated into theoretical frameworks that provide context for how to evaluate measurements in ways that provide predictive capability, Plant said. Moreover, the ecosystem of cell therapy product development in regenerative medicine is expansive, comprising multi-scale, dynamic, complex systems nested within each other (see Figure 1-1). Identifying the theoretical approaches that will bring these disparate data together in the appropriate context must be addressed. A systems approach is needed to analyze large-scale data from various sources (e.g., omics data, clinical indicators, starting materials) and begin to contextualize it using modeling frameworks, said Plant (see Figure 1-2). If one has not identified which measurements capture a product's critical quality attributes, it will be impossible to identify the critical manufacturing process parameters that are required to achieve those CQAs.

In addition to a focus on data, data structures, data modeling, and how data modeling and theory can help cultivate the understanding and development of regenerative medicine products, Roy encouraged workshop participants to consider several additional issues. In particular, he mentioned challenges related to data-intensive analytical methods and theoretical models, strategies to influence the regulatory process using data and theoretical approaches, and the use of systems modeling and artificial intelligence to optimize and manage the complex supply chain for regenerative medicine products. He asked participants to consider best practices for data sharing, data collection, and clinical trial design (e.g., collecting longitudinal data from patients) to enable systems thinking across the regenerative medicine ecosystem. Other considerations he mentioned related to strategies in education and workforce development to prepare the next generation of scientists, technicians, and leaders to understand big data and systems thinking.

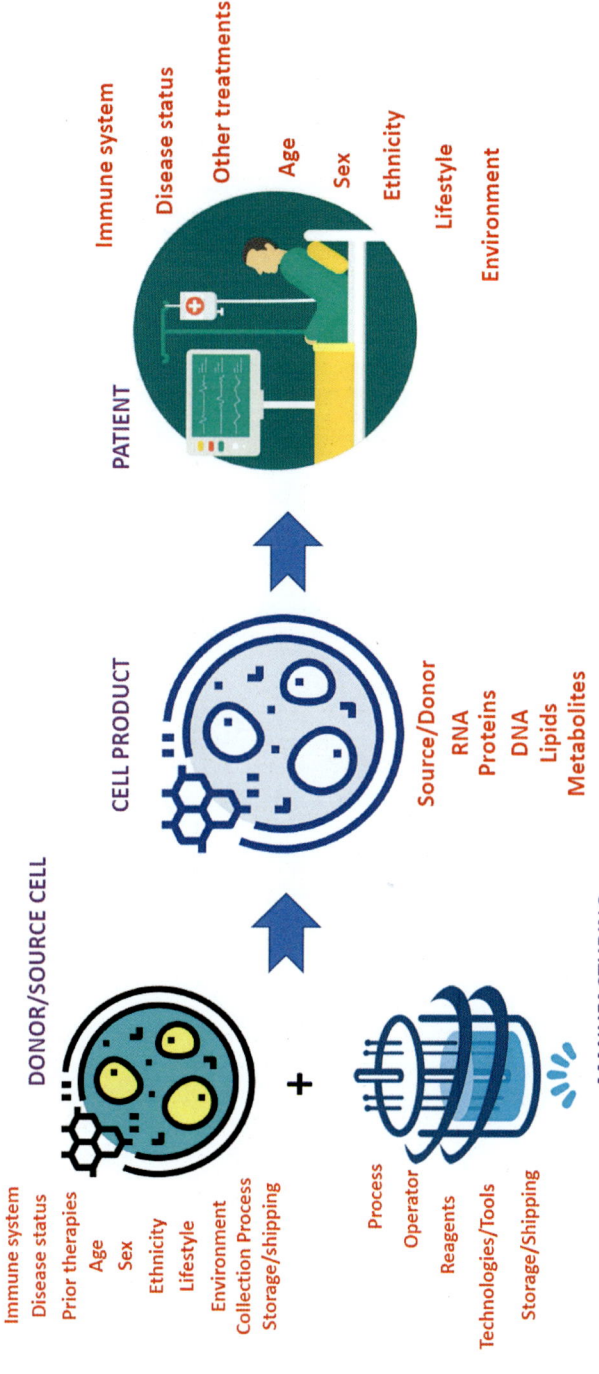

FIGURE 1-1 Cell therapy: interaction of multi-scale dynamic complex systems.
SOURCE: Krishnendu Roy workshop presentation, October 22, 2020.

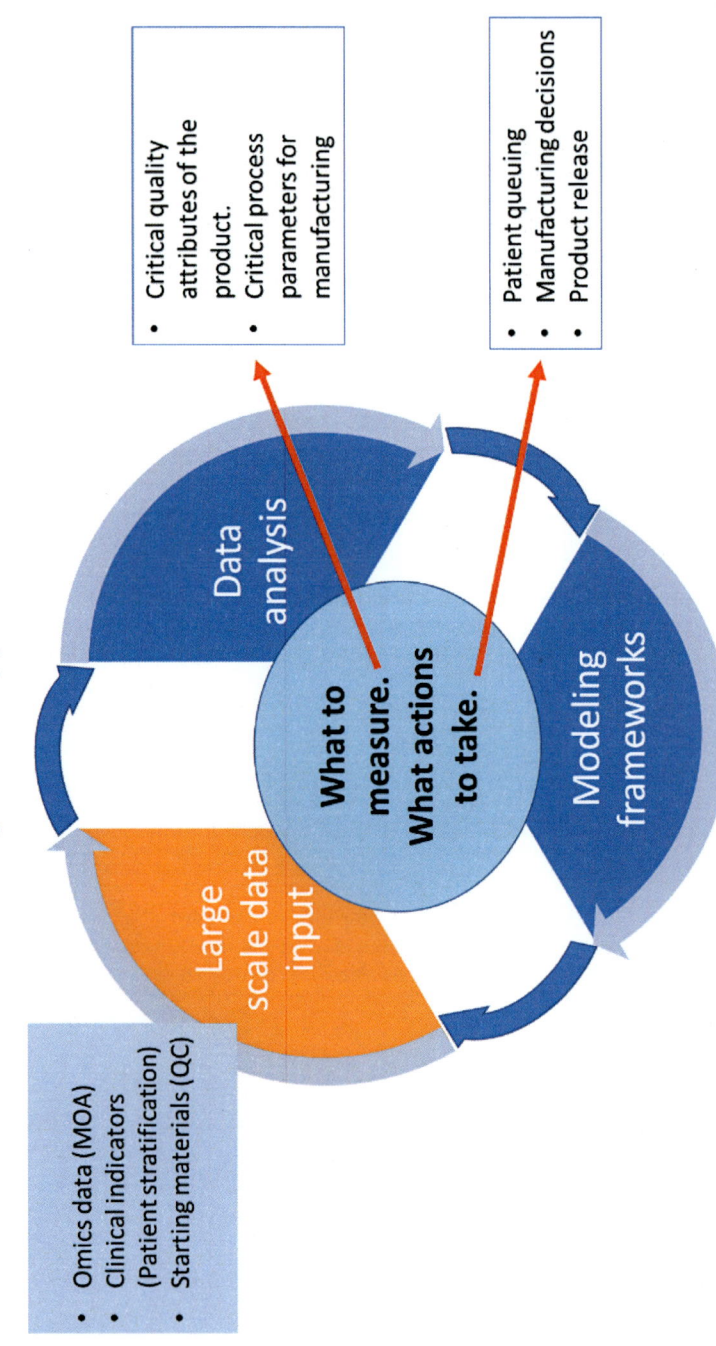

FIGURE 1-2 A systems approach to inform the regenerative medicine field.
NOTE: MOA = mechanism of action; QC = quality control.
SOURCE: Anne Plant workshop presentation, October 22, 2020.

ORGANIZATION OF THE PROCEEDINGS

This Proceedings of a Workshop summarizes the presentations and discussions that took place at the workshop on October 22–23, 2020. The first session provided an introduction to systems thinking concepts (Chapter 2). Speakers discussed systems thinking, its application to the development of regenerative medicine, and computational approaches for systems-level data collection. The second session explored the role of systems thinking in addressing challenges related to CQAs (Chapter 3). It included a fireside chat on systems thinking and the regulation of regenerative medicine products as well as a panel discussion on the costs of not implementing systems thinking approaches. The third session looked at challenges associated with data collection, aggregation, and sharing (Chapter 4). Its presentations examined data challenges with omics analysis and disease modeling, the use of big data for clinical stratification of patents, and opportunities to use large datasets to predict patient outcomes. The fourth session focused on challenges and opportunities associated with systems-level analysis and modeling (Chapter 5). Speakers discussed the development of algorithms for single-cell genomics, strategies for modeling dynamic data to identify a reduced variable space, and the adoption of metabolic modeling tools in the biopharmaceutical industry. The fifth session considered strategies to address regenerative medicine manufacturing and supply chain challenges with systems-level approaches (Chapter 6). Speakers discussed the use of artificial intelligence in cell and gene therapies, modeling the manufacturing process in regenerative medicine, and supply chain and cost modeling. The sixth session explored issues in workforce development related to systems thinking (Chapter 7). Panelists in that session discussed challenges and opportunities for training and workforce development in data science, artificial intelligence, and computational biology.

2

Introduction to Systems Thinking Concepts

Important Points Highlighted by Individual Speakers

- Bottom-up, mechanistic, linear, causation-driven approaches to understanding macro-level behavior of biological systems are limited when considering complex systems. Barriers to implementing top-down, system-level approaches include multi-scale systems, dynamics, heterogeneity, feedback control, and non-linearity. (Bialek, Huang, Zandstra)
- Bottom-up, reductionist hypotheses and approaches can lead to a proliferation of parameters; this challenge can potentially be addressed by applying top-down, system-level principles. (Bialek)
- Underlying molecular structures and mechanisms need to be integrated into critical quality attributes and other measurements to move the field of cell therapy from empirical mechanistic modeling toward process development. (Zandstra)
- Systems thinking can be used to predict macroscopic phenomena while bypassing the need to explicitly unmask all the quantitative dynamics operating at the microscopic level. (Huang)
- A common challenge with cell reprogramming is inefficiency due to the generation of many different cell types or cells that do not respond. A systems-level perspective may be needed to better understand the cellular response to reprogramming, and how to encourage cells to move to the desired state. (Huang)
- Engineering design approaches can be used to address some of the barriers in the field of regenerative medicine in order to improve the products that are produced for patients. (Zandstra)

The first session of the workshop offered an introduction to systems thinking concepts with the aims of providing important background to systems thinking approaches and related terminology and exploring specific examples of how systems thinking has been applied in areas of health and medicine, including potential opportunities in the regenerative medicine space. The session was moderated by Claudia Zylberberg of Akron Biotech and featured presentations that described how systems thinking can be applied to the development of regenerative medicines and that explored computational approaches for systems-level data collection.

AN INTRODUCTION TO SYSTEMS THINKING

The speakers in this session discussed how to define systems thinking. The simplest way to define the systems perspective is to contrast it with the reductionist perspective, said William Bialek, the John Archibald Wheeler/Battelle Professor in Physics at Princeton University and the Visiting Presidential Professor of Physics at the Graduate Center of the City University of New York. The reductionist perspective focuses on identifying microscopic components, with the implicit assumption that they can be used to reconstruct macroscopic phenomena. Systems-level thinking focuses on the macroscopic phenomena with a recognition that, while these phenomena ultimately originate from microscopic events, these macroscopic phenomena cannot be easily recreated or predicted using molecular components alone. The dualism between microscopic and macroscopic description distinguishes the two approaches, added Sui Huang, a professor at the Institute for Systems Biology. According to Peter Zandstra, the director of Michael Smith Laboratories and the director and a professor at the School of Biomedical Engineering at The University of British Columbia, conducting work across these scales requires researchers to adapt so that phenomena can be considered in a holistic manner. In his presentation, Bialek went on to provide an overview of systems thinking from his perspective as a theoretical physicist interested in biological problems.

Reductionist Hypotheses Do Not Imply Constructionist Hypotheses

Bialek described the enumeration of the molecular building blocks of life as among the great scientific triumphs of the 20th century. This process of molecular exploration has accelerated into the 21st century due to the ability to look at genome-wide phenomena rather than at single molecules at a time, he said. However, a long-standing problem faced by these efforts is that "the reductionist hypothesis does not imply a 'constructionist' one," in the words of physics Nobel laureate P. W. Anderson in a seminal paper (Anderson, 1972, p. 393). That is, the mere identification

INTRODUCTION TO SYSTEMS THINKING CONCEPTS 11

of all building blocks of a system is not tantamount to understanding how to put those pieces back together and to recover the behavior of interest at a macroscopic level. Anderson emphasized conceptual concerns about the relationships among the different sciences, but these issues have practical implications for understanding living systems as well.

Example from Early Fruit Fly Development

To illustrate these implications, Bialek described a biological process that is controlled by a genetic network and considered what can be predicted if all the relevant genes and their interactions have been identified. In the process, many of these genes encode transcription factors that regulate the expression of other genes in the network. A situation in which some genes shape the expression of other genes is not hypothetical, he said, and could describe many biological processes, even in mammalian cells. A classic example of a process controlled by a genetic network is found in early events in the development of a fruit fly, which provided one of the first opportunities to identify all the relevant molecules in a defined biological process. In fruit flies, development occurs along the long axis of the embryo (see Figure 2-1). Female fruit flies generate oocytes (developing eggs) that have crucial molecules serving as developmental landmarks (Alberts et al., 2002). The molecules create morphogen gradients that result in the definition of the anterior, posterior, and other larval structures in the future embryo. The molecules control gene expression, either directly—as transcription factors—or indirectly, as signaling molecules. These molecules are called "gap" genes, as the absence of a gap gene will result in a gap in the body plan of the embryo. These gap genes feed into a set of molecules called "pair-rule" genes, and the striped patterns of pair-rule expression provide a blueprint for the segmented body plan of the fully developed organism. Fruit flies are a particularly useful organism in which to monitor these processes in the laboratory, Bialek said. The transition from maternal effect genes (or maternal inputs) to pair-rule genes occurs in just 3 hours, and after 24 hours the egg hatches and the larva crawls away.

Proliferation of Parameters

All of the molecules involved in this process of fruit fly development have been identified, and the mechanisms represented by arrows in Figure 2-1 have also begun to be understood, Bialek said. However, identifying all the relevant genes and their interactions in a network is not sufficient for developing a model that can make quantitative predictions, due to the proliferation of parameters. For instance, each of the large blue arrows in Figure 2-1 has multiple parameters attached to it. For an arrow that

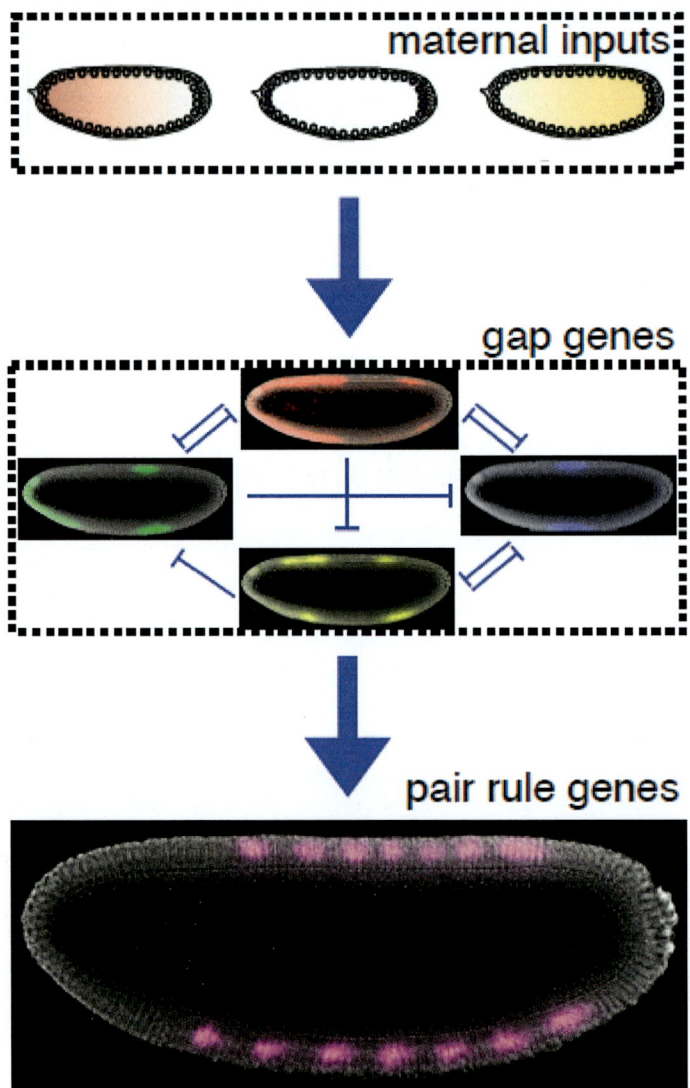

FIGURE 2-1 Fruit fly early development: from maternal inputs to larva.
SOURCES: William Bialek workshop presentation, October 22, 2020. Images adapted from Petkova et al., 2019.

represents a single transcription factor controlling the expression level of another gene, then the relevant associated parameters include the concentration at which the effect of that control process is half-maximal (i.e., the threshold for "turning things on") and the sharpness of that threshold. When two or more arrows converge, there is even more hidden complexity, describing how those signals combine; in principle, this could be an arbitrarily complex function. Given that four genes and three inputs are involved in this process, there are 28 possible arrows and thus more than 50 different parameters, Bialek said. Thus, creating a model of early fruit fly development with predictive power would require knowing what numbers to assign to all 50 or more parameters. Even in the well-studied case of fruit fly development, these numbers remain unknown. This is one very practical example in which even after one has carried out the reductionist work of identifying all of the constituent parts of a system, it is not necessarily possible to predict the behavior of that system as a whole from knowing the isolated behavior of its component parts.

Adding Systems-Level Ideas to the Reductionist Description

The variety of reactions to this problem of proliferation of parameters can be used, roughly, to classify the work being done in the field from different perspectives, including physics and systems biology, Bialek said. For instance, one approach is to concede that systems are so complicated that "quantitative biology" is really about learning complex models from limited data. Additional approaches, Bialek said, hold that (1) the only hope for a real theory is evolution (i.e., it is not about how things are, but about how they are related historically); (2) not all parameters matter; or (3) although there are many parameters at the micro scale, emergent functional phenomena are simpler. Bialek focused on an approach to the proliferation of parameters that involves adding systems-level ideas to the reductionist description. This approach presumes there is some principle that, in effect, selects the parameters, rather than parameter choices being random. The entire system has some function in the life of the organism, and the idea is to have a mathematical characterization of this function that makes it possible to optimize performance at this function, in parallel with what is being selected for by evolution. In the extreme, the hypothesis that function has been optimized by evolution can be considered, which would circumvent the need to know all of the parameters.

Candidate Principle: Transmit as Much Relevant Information as Possible with Limited Resources

Bialek described an example of a candidate principle that may operate at the system level: transmit as much relevant information as possible with limited resources. In the simplest case, X → Y (where X = input and Y = output), the question is how much information does the output provide about the input? For example, for every cell in an embryo to decide what body part it will become in the final pattern, it needs information about where it is located within the embryo. Each cell has an enormous amount of information and knows where it is to 1 percent accuracy, Bialek said. This level of precision is evident in cells' positioning and the precision with which developmental events are reproducible between embryos. In the case of fruit flies, for instance, at just 3 hours into development there are fewer than 100 rows of cells along the length of the embryo, so that 1 percent precision means that every cell knows where it is, he said. A challenge in trying to "squeeze all of the information" out of these signaling molecules is that they are present at such low concentrations that any measurements of those concentrations will be noisy (variable due to a range of extrinsic or intrinsic factors). Squeezing out as much information as possible can be done in a mathematically precise way, Bialek said.

In considering how much information inputs and outputs provide about each other, it may seem as if the information cannot be more precise or accurate, particularly if the output is a noisy version of the input, Bialek said. However, that information does not depend exclusively on the noise level; it also depends on the distribution of signals moving through this input–output device. If the concentrations of the input molecules are always very low and the input-output device only turns on at a high concentration, then the device would always be off and no information would be transmitted, regardless of the noise level. Therefore, squeezing as much information through the system as possible depends on matching the input–output relationship, the noise level, and the distribution of inputs. These ideas date back to research done decades ago on vision, in which Laughlin argued that the input–output relationships of neurons in the fly retina were actually matched to the distribution of input light intensities that the insect encounters as it flies through the world (Laughlin, 1981). More generally, with fixed input/output relationship and noise, information can be maximized by adjusting the distribution of inputs ("achieving capacity") or, with fixed noise and limited dynamic range at the output, information can be maximized by adjusting the mean input–output relation. This "matching" is a parameter-free prediction. In some cases, the neurons may require adaptation mechanisms that have not yet been identified but, more broadly, the adaptation phenomena that have already been identified in the nervous system can be understood as accomplishing this kind of match.

Applying Parameter-Free Prediction to Genetic Regulatory Elements

Bialek returned to the early development of the fruit fly to explore the application of this type of parameter-free prediction to genetic regulatory elements. It is possible to conduct experiments to simultaneously measure the concentrations of one of the input molecules in every cell (i.e., the maternal signals) as well as the concentrations of one of the output or intermediate molecules (i.e., the gap genes), which reveals a sigmoidal relationship on average (Gregor et al., 2007). Because this work involves thousands of samples drawn from the relative probability distributions, it is possible to characterize the noise in the system in addition to the input–output relationship. Bialek discussed how to determine whether an input–output device that has this relationship between input concentration and output concentration—as well as this level of noise—transmits as much information as possible. Adjusting the distribution of input concentrations to push as much information through as possible—implementing the principle outlined above—becomes a numerical problem with no free parameters. This approach predicts the distribution of inputs but is more sensitive to the distribution of outputs, which is predicted to have a double-peaked form, but with some occupation of the intermediate levels, and this prediction is in good quantitative agreement with experiments (Tkačik et al., 2008). Bialek described this as one of the first indications that this vision of collecting information based on inputs and outputs made sense and that different aspects of the data are related to one another.

The next step along this path is to determine how to deal with more complex systems, which have multiple inputs and outputs, Bialek said. In the fly embryo, for example, the relevant information is not the morphogen concentration, but rather the position of cells in the embryo (Dubuis et al., 2013). Thus, tracing back to information about position yields more predictions about how the system should behave. Unfolding these ideas can make more explicit the algorithms needed to read out the information that is encoded in the various levels of expression. Including all the gap genes eliminates the ambiguities and recovers the 1 percent precision described above. This work can be tested using fruit fly genetics by observing mutants in which some maternal inputs have been deleted, Bialek added. Mutants defective in maternal inputs produce distorted patterns of gap gene expression. These algorithms can be used to read where a cell "thinks" it is in a mutant and then predict where pair-rule stripes should be, quantitatively and with no free parameters (Petkova et al., 2019).

Possible Advances Using Top-Down Principles

Injecting top-down, system-level principles can generate detailed, quantitative predictions, thus circumventing highly parameterized bottom-up models, Bialek said. However, a challenge with this approach is the inverse of the challenge raised by Anderson. That is, the most powerful experimental tools are microscopic: they are able to probe and manipulate biological systems at the molecular level, not the system level. It is clear that the bottom-up approach cannot be used all the way up to the system level. Moving forward with this approach, Bialek said, will require investigating whether these top-down principles can be used to reach all the way down to the molecular level.

APPLYING SYSTEMS THINKING TO THE DEVELOPMENT OF REGENERATIVE MEDICINES

In his presentation Zandstra provided two examples as a way to explore the application of systems thinking to the development of regenerative medicines in various contexts, ranging from translational problems to therapeutic applications.

Growing Blood Stem Cells as Therapies for Leukemia

Zandstra's first example was centered on the work of growing blood stem cells as therapies for leukemia. This field was shaped by early discoveries and foundational observations published in the 1960s about how stem cells relate to their differentiated progeny and how a system—such as a distributed hematopoietic system—could be regulated through feedback control (Till et al., 1964). This example, Zandstra said, serves as a reminder that the foundation of systems biology and its use in regenerative medicine (i.e., stem cell biology) was established through observations and mathematical modeling conducted by physicists and hematologists who were seeking to understand cells. Specifically, Till and colleagues looked at how cells form colonies, investigated the properties of those colonies, and explored how components of the system interacted with one another to explain the responses of those colonies to transplantation and other processes. One of the early observations in this work was the potential role of feedback control in the cell creation system. This insight led to an investigation into why it is so difficult to grow blood stem cells when different cell types are generated that are continuously influencing their growth and differentiation. An empirical solution was developed by matching the rates of media addition and dilution of these cultures to the rates of secretion of inhibitory factors, which had a positive effect on the ex vivo expansion of blood stem cells (Csaszar et al., 2012). However, Zandstra said, this approach did not provide an understanding of the complexity in the system represented by various molecules being secreted at varying rates either in static or "fed-batch" systems. Further work by Kirouac et al. (2010) elaborated on the structure and parametrization of the communication networks behind this feedback.

From Empirical to Mechanistic Modeling in Cell Therapy Process Development

Zandstra said that to move the field of cell therapy from empirical mechanistic modeling toward process development, the underlying molecular structures and mechanisms need to be integrated and considered as part of a larger model. This will require careful consideration about how those structures and mechanisms are integrated with the critical quality attributes (e.g., identity, purity, potency) and the measurements taken during these cultures[1] (Lipsitz et al., 2016). The intent, he said, is to move from completely empirical approaches to optimizing systems toward using more relevant data to define systems. In the context of a human stem cell–centric cell–cell communication network in which there are secreted factors in the system, this approach can be used to help elucidate which cells are secreting which factors, the directionality of these factors, and the overall function of the system when the factors are used to modulate the interaction networks. One example of research using an integrated systems approach involved the use of omics technologies to associate cell types within the hematopoietic system with certain molecules (Qiao et al., 2014). These molecules are associated with pathways, and those pathways are associated with effects, thus allowing for a reductionist representation of the cell communication network. Researchers then began to investigate those properties of the system that could be manipulated to change different aspects of the network (Caldwell et al., 2015). By rebalancing the network according to receptor expression, compartmentalization, and other methods of changing feedback via molecular components as well as overall niche components within the system, Zandstra and colleagues were able to generate next-generation bioreactors (Csaszar et al., 2014). These bioreactors can then be used to take baseline measurements of a cell culture system, measure key factors within the system, then control—in an automated fashion—the way media are added and the types of components that are added to the media. Using this approach has had a positive effect on the ability to grow total cells and

---

[1] These measurements can include the gene expression signature of input cells, the fraction of proliferative T cell subtypes, cytokine activity, metabolite biomarker levels, and the pH rate of change.

progenitor cells, he added. Zandstra's team has since implemented structures that underpin some of these bioreactor systems within clinical production processes for expanding blood stem cells. At the time of the workshop, more than 50 patients had been treated with expansion systems based, in part, on this fed-batch-based approach[2] (Cohen et al., 2020).

Generating Immunotherapies from Pluripotent Stem Cells

Zandstra used his second example, the generation of immunotherapies from pluripotent stem cells, to highlight a challenge in this field. The aim of the stem cell–derived manufacturing of immunotherapies is to move toward a universal, homogenous, and scalable off-the-shelf product. This is a challenging endeavor, Zandstra said, because generating mature T cells from stem cells involves a long and complex differentiation process: from pluripotent stem cells, either in their normal or engineered state, to blood progenitor cells, to progenitor T cells, and eventually to more mature T cells. One approach to this process is to develop technologies to control these various phases, which entails high degrees of complexity in terms of the timing, dosing, and types of molecules that are applied during the differentiation process. These factors likely control which types of progeny are produced from the progenitor T cells, including effector, regulatory, and other types of T cells in the system.

Computational Systems Modeling for the Predictive Design of T Cell Therapies

Zandstra explained that two signaling pathways are especially important in the process that differentiates pluripotent stem cells into various types of mature T cells: (1) Notch activation, which is necessary early on but must decrease as the cell moves toward T cell maturation, and (2) T cell receptor (TCR)-based signaling, which is eventually important for the proliferation and maturation of T cells. A major question is how to design environments that can control systems that involve such complex and multi-step processes (e.g., by quantitatively modulating Notch and TCR signaling to match in vivo thymopoiesis [the process by which thymocytes, a type of immune cell present in the thymus, are transformed into mature T cells]). Zandstra and his colleagues are working in this area at three different levels:

---

[2]Fed-batch processes are partly open systems that involve intermittent or continuous feeding of nutrients. This approach can result in higher cell growth and product formation (Lim and Shin, 2013).

1. Mass action kinetics-based modeling of Notch-DLL4 signaling to explore how to quantitatively control biochemical pathways driving T cell fate;
2. Cell population modeling of thymopoiesis to understand how culture parameters modulate cell T cell differentiation and kinetics; and
3. Cellular kinetic pharmacokinetic/pharmacodynamic modeling to investigate how culture-generated T cell populations interact with human (patho-)physiology.

The first of these approaches seeks to achieve a basic understanding of the mass-action kinetics behind the signaling pathways that are activated by identifying the key signaling moieties that can be measured during the process. The second approach is related to cell population modeling and is similar to work within the hematopoietic system. This approach attempts to understand what factors—whether known or yet to be discovered from omics data—can be applied to guide the differentiation process. The third approach focuses on relating the key properties of cells measured in vitro to the overall biology of those cells in vivo, ideally in the patient. The systems pharmacology aspects of cell therapy products are still poorly understood, Zandstra added.

Zandstra went on to describe how Notch- and TCR-signaling models can be used for in silico bead design and optimization in order to look at the relationship between various signaling activation complexes on the surface of a progenitor cell and techniques that affect cell differentiation. In this endeavor the goal is to determine how signaling parameters affect cell differentiation. He noted that it is important to match the needs of the differentiation system with the signaling timing and processes that are under way.

Zandstra also presented a second example of how cellular kinetic pharmacokinetic/pharmacodynamic modeling can be used to understand the cellular properties underlying clinical response. As indicated by data on the signal of the chimeric antigen receptor (CAR) T cells in patients as a function of different patient examples, a major challenge is that clinical CAR T cell pharmacokinetic and exposure-response relationships are highly variable (Mueller et al., 2018). As a result, it has been difficult to understand what properties of cells should be measured to make predictions about the persistence of CAR T cells and their effects on tumors. By applying more complex models to processes that have developmental programs involving various T cell populations (e.g., naïve-memory T cells, effector T cells), it is possible to begin to simulate and extract from these models the parameters that may have the greatest ability to predict tumor mass reduction. As more data become available, the model's ability to make relevant predictions can be improved; this will feed back into informing the quality attributes around which cell cultures are designed and the ideal profiles of the cell therapy.

Applying Engineering Design Principles to Overcome Barriers in Cell Therapy Translation

There are opportunities to move the field forward by applying engineering design principles to overcome barriers in cell therapy translation, said Zandstra (Tewary et al., 2018). In the future, he said, it would be helpful to consider the point at which the systems component of mathematical modeling begins to extend beyond simple empirical models to more complex mechanistic models and, ultimately, to the types of emergent models discussed by Bialek. In such emergent models, the degree of complexity is so great that strategies are needed to extract key governing principles from those datasets. These techniques can be applied to understand, predict, and, eventually, control the cycle that underlies both discovery and translation, Zandstra added. Furthermore, these approaches could be applied to deal with some of the barriers faced in the field of regenerative medicine: for example, multi-scale aspects of systems, dynamics, heterogeneity, and the nonlinearity that is typically due to feedback control and other interactions within the models. Addressing those barriers, he said, has the potential to substantially improve the types of products that are produced for patients.

SYSTEMS DYNAMICS OF CELL-STATE TRANSITIONS: RELEVANCE FOR REGENERATIVE MEDICINE

Huang presented an exploration of systems dynamics of cell-state transitions and their relevance for regenerative medicine, with a focus on single-cell transcriptomics.

Cell Type Reprogramming as Cell-State Transition

Cell type reprogramming is a core process of interest throughout the field of regenerative medicine, Huang said. Researchers often seek to reprogram cells from one type to another through some form of manipulation; for example, transitioning induced pluripotent stem (iPS) cells into a particular type of neuron or transitioning pancreas α cells into pancreas β cells, which are useful for diabetes treatment. However, this vision is currently not fully aligned with reality, he said. In attempting to manipulate the cells in multicellular organisms with the intention of creating a desired cell type, a cell may be subjected to some intervention that can instead result in a variety of undesired cells. This is a problem for regenerative medicine: not just the low rate of cells that respond ("failure to push hard enough"), but also the generation of many different cell types ("failure to channel") is at the heart of the notorious inefficiency of any reprogramming manipulation. A systems perspective is needed in order to understand why this diversification happens, which cell types will be generated, and how to "herd" all the cells into the desired direction, he said.

Huang elaborated on the problem with the traditional, reductionist understanding of the process of cell type reprogramming as "molecular causation," which is evident in models that consider a certain protein to cause a certain effect or phenotype. Using such causative pathway models, researchers try to block or stimulate proteins in order to prevent or promote the effect. This type of linear, molecular causation-based thinking is common across the biological sciences, he said, but it is not the appropriate perspective with which to approach this problem. From a stricter, formal standpoint it is more appropriate to consider the process in terms of a state transition, whereby some state (Cell Type 1) changes (i.e., transitions) to another state (Cell Type 2). For instance, through the process of state transition, a stem cell may become a differentiated cell, or a fibroblast may become an iPS cell. Within this perspective, the manipulation is intended to trigger the cell-state transition. This requires defining the state of the cell, which is governed by the gene regulatory network which has evolved to generate cell states and cell types.

Within the genome, every gene has some level of expression based on its profile, but the individual genes in the network are interdependent rather than independent with respect to altering their expression, Huang said. Changing the state of a cell changes the gene expression profile, but how individual genes contribute to this collective change is dictated by the network. The interactions within the network cannot be changed. Ultimately, what changes is not the network, but the state of the network with respect to the expression level of the individual genes that it contains. The network is hard-wired, but it changes its state as defined by the profile of the expression level of the genes. Since the genes are interdependent, some gene expression profiles are more likely to be realized (more stable) than others. Therefore, Huang explained, all possible gene expression profiles can be mapped to a sort of "potential landscape" in which the "elevation" crudely represent the probability of a given gene expression profile being realized. The potential wells (valleys) are the *attractor states*, which are the stable, observable gene expression profiles that fully satisfy the gene interaction rules imposed by the network (Chang et al., 2008; Huang et al., 2005; Zhou et al., 2012). The complex gene network of a genome generates multiple attractor states, a phenomenon called multi-stability. Each attractor is a cell type. Huang likened the study of transitions between attractor states to Waddington's study of the epigenetic landscapes (Waddington, 1957).

Waddington attempted to frame development as a process that takes place on a landscape where the network seeks natural states (the valleys). This metaphor explains developmental robustness, discreteness of cell types, and instabilities that impose cell fate decisions, which are represented by the watersheds. Huang suggested that it would be valuable to apply this basic conceptual idea to regenerative medicine.

Complications to the Model of Cell-State Transitions

Huang described two complications to cell-state transitions within multicellular organisms with populations of millions of cells. Because of stochastic fluctuations, or non-genetic heterogeneity, these cells are all slightly different—even within a clonal cell population. Single-cell transcriptomics allows for a precise view of individual cells, while big data and statistical data analysis allow for individual cells to be plotted in a reduced dimensional space, creating clusters of various cells in various states. However, these individuated clusters, or subpopulations of cells, must be related to a theory that explains how a finite number of allowed attractor states can emerge from the gene regulatory network. Huang discussed novel advances in single-cell transcriptomes that are helping to advance this work. Traditionally, gene expression profiles are created by taking the entire population of millions of cells as one sample (e.g., by triggering differentiation and measuring gene expression across the entire cell culture), thus using population averages to study transcriptomes. However, by using single-cell-resolution measurements, a matrix can be generated in which each column is a cell, and each row is a gene. Single-cell resolution analysis can be used to perturb differentiation that changes the cell population structure, allowing changes in the cell–gene matrix to be observed instead of using an aggregate measure of the gene expression profile.

Another complication arises due to continued branching into various cell types, which may either be desired or undesired cell types. In the linear conception of such a process, a cell begins at some state, and a signal or intervention results in the change to a desired state. However, in a nonlinear process an intervention or signal may result in various and often polar-opposite states. Because cell-state changes are nonlinear, it is necessary to consider, beyond mere linear causation, the stability/instability/multi-stability of cell states. In addition, Huang said, the heterogeneity or stochasticity arising from each cell being in a slightly different state must be considered because those different cell states result in instability. To illustrate, Huang presented an animated model demonstrating the processes associated with cell-state changes. In order to transition between attractor states, the state space must be destabilized, which leads to a critical transition point at which the cell's attractor state is flattened. With this destabilization comes an element of uncontrollability. During the transitional cell states, some cells will move to the desired direction of the cell-state space, but others will move in aberrant directions toward an undesired outcome. This dispersion is reflected in single-cell analysis. The positions of individual cells in such analyses are governed by the underlying landscape which represents the constraints from the gene regulatory network. Stable clusters in these analyses represent the manifestation of the constraints of more and less stable states (i.e., the shape of the single-cell clusters and their changes reflect the dynamics on the epigenetic landscape).

Regarding the spontaneous branching of cell states, Huang said that after the cell state is destabilized, the cells disperse and hence become more different, which is readily measurable by single-cell gene expression analysis: the destabilization reduces the correlation between those cells. While this loss of correlation between the cells is intuitive to researchers in the field, what is more interesting is that in the same single-cell expression data matrix, the genes start to correlate with each other, Huang said. In summary, single-cell resolution measurement exposes destabilization and can be used to predict an impending bifurcation or "tipping point," Huang said. At the transition, when maximally destabilized, just before the tipping point, the correlation between cell states will decrease while the correlation between genes will increase. By contrast, in the attractor state cells are maximally correlated (because they are forced to be in essentially the same state) while genes are uncorrelated (because the sole source of departure from the "set-point" expression level of a gene for each cell, imposed by the attractor state, is gene expression noise) (Mojtahedi et al., 2016).

Huang presented an example in which researchers attempted to differentiate iPS cells into cardiomyocytes (Trachana et al., 2018). In order to do this, it is necessary to transition cells along a particular path. As mentioned earlier, the practical challenge is overcoming the inefficiency of achieving directed differentiation, because some cells are lost to the wrong fate (Palpant et al., 2015). In this case, cells undergo two critical state transitions in the move from epiblast to primitive streak state, and they can arrive at various states that may or may not be desirable (Bargaje et al., 2017). Measuring cell–cell correlation reveals that in the move to the first jump, the cell–cell correlation decreases. However, in the same process, increasing numbers of gene-pairs suddenly start to correlate, suggesting a critical transition. The specific genes that correlate are important in this transition, as predicted by the theory: they are the ones that in the gene regulatory circuit regulate each other (hence correlate or anti-correlate with each other) and therefore likely are the genes that play central roles in driving the transition. However, there are also undesired cells that appear, which in this case are the endodermal lineages as opposed to the mesodermal lineages that lead to the cardiomyocytes. This is the reason why reprogramming into a desired cell type is so inefficient, Huang said.

Huang emphasized that, in terms of systems thinking, the gene regulatory network that governs a gene expression profile as well as the quasi-potential (i.e., "epigenetic") landscape and critical transitions (i.e., bifurcation) are important factors. The theory of such landscapes—and the measurements of cell–cell and gene–gene correlation explained previously—describes how individual states are more or less stable (relatively), especially with many cell types in a single population. Typical flow cytometry initially depicts just one dimension of the high-dimensional dynamics involved in cell transitions; however, single-cell data can elucidate high-dimensional dynamic states.

DISCUSSION

Expanding Beyond Empirical Modeling

Referring to an earlier remark by Zandstra that the systems component of mathematical modeling is becoming more than the mere application of empirical models, Zylberberg asked about the point at which the complexity becomes so great that key principles need to be extracted from datasets. This question is still being explored, Zandstra said, as researchers work to discover how to extract measurable parameters from global observations of cell states. The parameters may not be the identity of a molecule, but rather some combination of factors, including molecule, time, and perhaps some measure of concentration level. Together, a set of parameters could provide more information about a system than any individual measurement of a molecular state. While this is still a challenging area of study, there is progress being made toward understanding how a combination of parameters may offer insight into how those factors can influence different outcomes within culture systems, Zandstra said.

Noise in Biological Systems

Noise is important to consider because it can present an important challenge in understanding biological systems, Bialek said. He offered the analogy of an amplifier and speaker to demonstrate the concerns related to noise in a system. The output of an amplifier can be very noisy, despite the amplifier itself being nearly noiseless. In such a case, the noise may be created by a high-gain input that is being amplified. In the biological context, if concentrations of molecules are low, then all of the processes will be noisy—this is a feature of the physics or physical chemistry of the cell. What is unique in biological processes is that, for some reason, cells' fates are entrusted to a small number of molecules. This is a surprise, Bialek said, and operating in this regime makes the cells' jobs difficult. Perhaps, he continued, much of what happens in the cell is shaped by the evolutionary choice to operate in this regime where noise plays such an important role. The presence of noise in the system does not reflect intrinsic sloppiness, he added.

In translational research and regenerative medicine development, it is sometimes difficult to distinguish between noise and a poorly specified system, Zandstra said. This can result in a poor understanding of key system parameters or an inappropriate technological design that is ill-matched to the current level of understanding. He offered an example from the early research on pluripotent stem cells: the cells would be put in an undefined aggregate (an embryoid body), and the variability in the types of differentiation that emerged were considered to be partially due to system noise. It has since been discovered that the introduction of high concentrations of inductive molecules at certain stages will lead to more uniform and coordinated differentiation. This is not to say that noise is not a part of the underlying biological process of the cell fate divisions, Zandstra said. Rather, it means that systems can be designed to control the impact of the noise.

Obtaining Rates for T Cell Phenotypes in the Transit Model

With regard to how rates are obtained for the different T cell phenotypes in the transit model, many data are gathered from the baseline process in which genomic, single-cell, and cell-level information is collected, Zandstra said. There are hundreds—if not thousands—of parameters that could be measured within complex systems, but data cannot reasonably be collected for every potential parameter. The use of more abstract models has helped to determine where parameter sensitivity has the greatest impact. It is helpful to strike a balance between measuring parameters that are aligned with existing outputs and searching for instances in which they are not aligned, Zandstra added.

Similarities to Quality-by-Design

Some of the concepts discussed during the session, namely those related to controlling processes in order to reach a desired endpoint, sound similar to quality-by-design approaches used in the chemical medicine space, a workshop participant pointed out. The data presented by Bialek and Huang can be thought of as a cloud of information that falls in the design space of quality-by-design, Zandstra said. This makes it possible to consider how to map process parameters to that cloud. It also provides the flexibility to determine which cells are in the cloud and thus how parameter and process changes can be adapted while maintaining the desired attributes in cells. He suggested that this could provide a valuable opportunity to iterate faster around product development.

Choosing Targets Within Cell Systems

Addressing the issue of which attractor states are best for clinical efficacy in patients, Huang drew a distinction within the question between how researchers know which attractor cell to target (i.e., what kind of cell type is desired) and how these targets are realized. Referring to an example from his presentation, he described a situation where cardiomyocytes are desired but, in reality, a mixture of cell types would be needed due to the highly dynamic nature of cells. For example, in tumor therapy, in most cases one cannot simply kill tumor cells; it is necessary to account for other dynamics of tissues and tumors. Many cell types interact with other cell types, which presents a challenge for researchers. They must choose not only which attractor state to target, but also the distribution of millions of cells among different attractors that is necessary for cells to communicate with each other. If some cell-organizing principle were discovered in the future, it could make it possible to circumvent the need to understand every detail; instead it would be possible to simply trigger a process to keep development on the right path.

The history of models in developmental biology, Bialek said, began with Turing's focus on how cells communicate and on the patterns emerging from those spatial interactions (Turing, 1952). The problem posed by Turing was how to make patterns form in the absence of any initial spatial inhomogeneities, but it was later appreciated that real embryos have "built in" spatial inhomogeneities. For example, a maternal effect gene at a particular place can drive every cell to make decisions, because it experiences a different concentration of the primary morphogen molecule. Consequently, the field bifurcated into one view that was dominated by a focus on interactions and another view that focused on cell autonomy. This bifurcation persists, in part, due to the nature of scientific experimentation. Disaggregating cells in order to study them individually makes it difficult to probe how they interact among each other. However, when cells are studied in aggregate, it is difficult to interrogate them individually—although there are now newer methods for studying cells together. Bialek suggested that once precision tools are available for interrogating individual cells in situ where their reactions can be probed, the two views may converge once again and demonstrate that the actual process contains elements of both conceptualizations. Discovering which organizing principles exist would be invaluable in revealing how those elements interact, he added.

Zandstra questioned how a network balancing within individual cells and the network structure may affect multi-scale tissue patterning. He and his colleagues recently made an initial effort to explore this issue at a simplistic level by looking at how rewiring in different levels of factors affects the Turing-like pattern events which occur in the simplest tissues.

Using Theory to Collect Data

Theory may be used not only to interpret data, but also to help reveal what types of data are most valuable to collect in order to build predictive models for cell-state conditions applied to cell therapies. Bialek commented that experimentation has a cyclical nature: some experiments spur theoretical insights that in turn raise new questions that can be investigated experimentally. The most interesting theoretical directions can depend on things that have not yet been measured, which drives researchers to return and make new measurements, Bialek said. For example, measuring the molecules in fly embryos at high precision is difficult, which discourages researchers from making such measurements unless they have some motivation or reason to think that a measurement at that level of precision would yield an interesting result. The question of how accurate a measurement needs to be is a theoretical one, Bialek said, because researchers are not generally inclined to collect measurements with greater precision than necessary just for the sake of doing so. While some questions are obvious to researchers even without a theory to motivate them, many of the details of experimental design—such as how many things need to be measured simultaneously, measurement accuracy, and the time resolution required to resolve transitions—are (or should be) informed by theory.

Theory plays a role in determining how precise measurements should be, Zylberberg added. Theory is at times purely academic, Huang said, noting that individuals may have unrealistic expectations for what theory can do. Theory offers a broad view, and it is generally beneficial for researchers to understand theory and then decide to what extent it will guide analysis. Currently, there is too much reliance on purely computational approaches, Huang said, but theory could be helpful to counteract this reliance, especially to the extent that it may reveal instances where it is not necessary to collect the fullest possible detail in terms of measurement.

Much of the session's discussion of systems had been related to cell engineering and decision making at the level of individual cells, Zylberberg noted. She posed a question to the panelists from an audience member about how the boundaries of a system are determined and asked whether there have been instances where the system had to be narrowed or broadened. System boundaries are drawn based on an inference that those boundaries will be productive, Bialek said, not on a belief that a system's interactions do not cross those boundaries. In the history of biology, Bialek said, progress has often been related to the degree to which processes being studied have been able to be isolated. For instance, in neuroscience that which is well understood is primarily related to situations in which one thing happens in one place. The less isolated that processes are, the more difficult it is to understand those processes. The drawing of boundaries is always considered, and such boundary drawing should be acknowledged as a component of the hypothesis itself. However, Bialek said, because boundaries are selected with the intent of making progress within those boundaries, one mode of failure may be the recognition that processes cross the boundaries too often for progress to be made within them. There is an iterative aspect to this process that is characteristic of all work on biological systems, he said. In some cases, such as in studying single molecules, the elements being studied are removed from their complex context in order to ensure that nothing goes in or out. In some ways this is productive, Bialek said, but in other ways it can sacrifice potentially important observations. Huang said that there is sometimes a dismissive attitude toward any work that is decontextualized. However, he pointed out that science must work through dissection. For instance, the heart could only be studied because scientists removed a heart from a dead body. This can be done operationally while still being aware of context, he noted.

Each type of entropy—Shannon, Tsallis, and Renyi—has its uses for capturing information,[3] Bialek said, but Shannon entropy corresponds to intuitions about what information means and is the same as the entropies familiar from physical chemistry, statistical mechanics, and other fields. Other entropies have value as well, in part because they are easier to estimate from finite data, making possible a broader range of connections between theory and experiment. However, on a conceptual basis, he said, Shannon entropy is privileged.

---

[3] For an overview of these different entropies, see Amigo et al. (2018).

3

Exploring the Challenges of Critical Quality Attributes: The Role of Systems Thinking

Important Points Highlighted by Individual Speakers

- In the field of regenerative medicine, a systems thinking approach can contribute to accelerating development and optimizing products by interrelating large-scale datasets on product characteristics (e.g., next-generation sequencing data), patients' clinical information (e.g., electronic health records), manufacturing, and delivery of care. (Abernethy)
- Challenges in applying systems thinking to regenerative medicine include the cost and complexity of linking multiple complex datasets from different sources to extract the relevant information, relatively low numbers of patients and products, and the need for a common language that enables stakeholders across disciplines to communicate and coordinate their efforts. (Abernethy)
- Systems thinking can be applied to therapeutic cell product development through an iterative process of integrating information about complex cell product characteristics with patient response data to identify the critical quality attributes of the cell product that should be monitored during good manufacturing practices. (Temple)
- The cell therapy manufacturing process is a system in and of itself, with interactions among its components. Measurements collected at each step of the process can be integrated with post-treatment patient information to adjust manufacturing parameters for more reliable, consistent, and efficient production. (Manian)

- Chimeric antigen receptor T cell therapies are evaluated using a systems biology approach that incorporates data from manufacturing, delivery, and patient outcomes into larger data analysis models. Single-cell omics analysis of patient heterogeneity in T cells can be used to understand how patient features affect critical product attributes and patient outcomes. (Bot)
- A consortium approach, including industry and academia, would advance the field of cell therapy and help optimize patient management by increasing the rate of durable responses and predicting or mitigating toxicities. (Bot)
- The consequences of not using a systems-level approach include failure of the translational research enterprise to deliver adequate understanding of product performance and beneficial therapy to patients (Temple), individualized patient-by-patient processes that are unaffordable to most of the population (Manian), and missed opportunities to expand the footprint of curative interventions (Bot).

During the second session of the workshop, presenters and attendees explored how systems thinking approaches may be applied to challenges associated with identifying the critical quality attributes in the discovery, regulation, and manufacturing of regenerative medicine. The session featured a fireside chat with Amy Abernethy, the principal deputy commissioner at the Food and Drug Administration (FDA), on the regulation of regenerative medicine products in the context of systems thinking approaches which was moderated by Anne Plant, a National Institute of Standards and Technology (NIST) Fellow and the former chief of the Biosystems and Biomaterials Division at NIST. Jane Lebkowski, the president of Regenerative Patch Technologies, moderated the subsequent panel discussion on the costs associated with not implementing systems thinking approaches. The panelists, who gave brief presentations as part of the panel included Adrian Bot, the vice president of translational medicine at Kite Pharma, Inc.; Bala Manian, the chief executive officer (CEO) of Mojave Bio, Inc.; Douglas Olson, the president and the CEO of Buhlmann Diagnostics Corp and a scientific advisory board member at Cell Manufacturing Technologies (CMaT); and Sally Temple, the scientific director, the principal investigator, and the co-founder of the Neural Stem Cell Institute. This session's objective was to understand the challenges associated with identifying critical quality attributes in the discovery, regulation, and manufacturing of regenerative medicine products and how systems thinking approaches may be applied.

SYSTEMS THINKING AND THE REGULATION OF REGENERATIVE MEDICINE PRODUCTS

Plant opened the session by noting that progress in the collection of large quantities of data, which is often omics-based, has made large datasets available for both biological and clinical sciences. As the development of advanced therapies becomes increasingly reliant on large datasets, it brings advantages as well as technical challenges in data collection, analysis, and the development of appropriate models to provide context to those data in order to provide predictive knowledge. Abernethy described opportunities and challenges associated with access to big data and systems thinking in the context of the regulatory landscape for regenerative medicine.

Systems Thinking and Large-Scale Data in the Regulatory Landscape

The conceptual approach of using large-scale datasets across the medical product development process—from early development to late-stage post-marketing evaluation—is of great importance to FDA, Abernethy said. An advantage of systems thinking is the opportunity to link various steps of the development process through datasets. This is helpful in characterizing products, understanding pharmacology and toxicology information, and discerning clinical effects. Using large-scale datasets to consider issues of efficacy, safety, and approval of drugs in the regenerative medicine space will help improve the quality of medical products, she said; however, despite great interest in using large-scale datasets to accelerate drug development, this is not yet a widespread practice.

Interrelating large-scale datasets of deep omics (deep learning applied to omics data) on the discovery side together with clinical data can support clinical evaluation. For example, Abernethy said, next-generation genomic sequencing data have been combined with electronic health record data to create appended datasets that marry those two types of information. In turn, those datasets could then be married with information about the manufacturing process of various regenerative therapies. Likewise, the datasets could be combined with information related to health care delivery. Combining these datasets can elucidate interrelated features across clinical development, quality manufacturing, and quality implementation on the health care delivery side. Furthermore, Abernethy said, this process can distinguish the issues of manufacturing and health care delivery that are more important to focus on from those that are of lesser consequence. However, the ability to gather seemingly disparate information by considering an entire set of interrelationships requires subject-matter expertise—not only in mathematics, but also in all of the different areas involved—to be able to understand the data in context. For FDA, this means developing the technical cross-checking capabilities needed to confirm findings. Thus, she said, there is much work to be done across the entire process.

Efforts to Combine Large-Scale Data Across the Wider Ecosystem of Components

Are there examples, Plant asked, of efforts that combine data over a wide ecosystem of components and then bring those data into the discovery, manufacturing, or delivery processes? Abernethy answered that these processes are not yet well-developed, but that some efforts are showing promise. For example, FDA is conducting a Model-Informed Drug Development pilot program[1] in which clinical pharmacologists, statisticians, and other FDA professionals are working with industry and drug developers to use preclinical and early clinical data to improve the planning of clinical trials, identify dosing more carefully, and predict the most consequential trial outcomes more accurately. Using information gathered from sources that historically were excluded from the trial design process, this process is increasing the knowledge used in the clinical trials context. Furthermore, essential preclinical safety models have been created to inform researchers as to what safety events might be seen in the clinical trial space. The pilot program, Abernethy said, is an important step in developing communication between regulators and the industry, and she suggested that a critical step in moving forward will be to create a common language to enable stakeholders to determine who is responsible for each step and how best to document datasets, methods, and outputs.

Work related to the coronavirus disease 2019 (COVID-19) is another area where researchers are intermarrying large datasets, Abernethy said. Computational modeling of repurposed drugs that have potential as therapeutics for COVID-19 is being overlaid with data from the use of those drugs in real clinical environments as well as with data about the risk of developing COVID-19. These data are being used to help identify potential drugs that can be repurposed as COVID-19 therapeutics and to determine priorities for clinical trials (Gordon et al., 2020). In the regenerative medicine space, long-term data are needed to better understand the long-term safety consequences of therapeutics. FDA issued guidance for cell and gene therapies in January 2020 that highlighted that the long-term safety consequences of gene therapies are not yet understood.[2] Preclinical models appended to

---

[1] More information about the Model-Informed Drug Development pilot program is available at https://www.fda.gov/drugs/development-resources/model-informed-drug-development-pilot-program (accessed December 8, 2020).

[2] FDA's cellular and gene therapy guidances are available at https://www.fda.gov/vaccines-blood-biologics/biologics-guidances/cellular-gene-therapy-guidances (accessed December 8, 2020).

clinical trials can inform what safety issues to monitor for, while follow-up information from insurance claims and electronic health records data can aid in better understanding longer-term clinical impacts, Abernethy added.

Shifting Dynamics in the Manufacturing Process

There is a push–pull dynamic in the manufacturing space, Plant said, between having a manufacturing process and then wanting to change, improve, or streamline that process, which may involve a change in starting materials. The philosophy of "product is the process" seems to have worked for some biological therapies, she said, but that philosophy may not apply as aptly to cell therapies, in which a philosophy of "product is the product" may be more appropriate. Will it shift the dynamic to have more data and a better understanding of what is important to measure in order to predict product success? she asked. Abernethy predicted that there will be continued movement in "product-is-the-process" thinking, especially in the regenerative medicine space with respect to n-of-1 or n-of-a-few therapies, which will require continued novel thinking and development.

Abernethy remarked that when she joined FDA in 2019, she discovered that the elements of the tightly controlled, professionalized manufacturing process were not specifically appended to an understanding of how patients perform. At that time, cross-linking manufacturing details and optimization details with electronic health records data went against common practice, she said. Currently, in late 2020, manufacturing plants are being built to include a series of intricate sensors. In the shift toward n-of-1 or n-of-a-few therapies, work is under way to interrelate details along the manufacturing pathway to clinical outcomes. This could help researchers explore the interrelationships among changes made to the manufacturing process, any resulting changes in the product, and the possible effects of those changes in people. Systems thinking, she added, provides an opportunity to think broadly about how different pieces can interrelate, given the tether of data and computation that is being created, and which can be used to understand the ripple effects.

Regulatory Challenges in Shifting Toward Systems Thinking

In shifting toward a systems thinking approach, Abernethy said, there are many areas FDA may need to address thoughtfully. For example, regulatory certainty is important for medical product development because it enables decisions about where to invest and it informs expectations along the pathway. Thus, FDA is cautious in making changes, as any shifts in FDA's approach have the potential to cause downstream effects on safety and effectiveness and to shift regulatory expectations in an environment in which people want certainty about what process to expect. Therefore, in exploring an area such as systems thinking and the interrelationship of multiple datasets, FDA would benefit from becoming more comfortable with the possible changes in the development frame. Efforts to link up various components are already ongoing in preclinical toxicity and post-marketing studies, she said, and she suggested that industry should also engage in this type of work.

FDA may also need to be able to clarify the characteristics of datasets, determine their fit for purpose, identify the appropriate analyses to enact for various tasks, and develop communication about those tasks, Abernethy said. Furthermore, different tasks are needed for various spaces. For instance, the specific tasks required in modeling preclinical toxicity and clinical trials differ from those involved in modeling to replace some part of the pathway. Familiarity with these different tasks can then enable the development of a set of prescribed events, such as guidance documents. For this multistep pathway Abernethy envisioned a series of pilots, such as the Model-Informed Drug Development pilot, along with those guidances for important components (e.g., conducting 15 years of follow-up research). Finally, she suggested that FDA should participate—either directly or via public–private partnerships—in projects to build regulatory familiarity, enabling regulators to develop the expertise required for this new approach.

Facilitating Systems Thinking Among FDA Sponsors

Is FDA planning, Plant asked, on taking any actions to facilitate systems thinking on the part of FDA sponsors? The Model-Informed Drug Development pilot is a good example of encouraging this shift, Abernethy replied. In the context of the current pandemic, FDA is participating in the COVID-19 Evidence Accelerator.[3] This set of activities is being conducted via a public–private partnership organized by the Reagan-Udall Foundation, FDA's congressionally mandated foundation. The Foundation has brought together stakeholders who have data—predominantly clinical data and real-world data relevant to COVID-19—and those willing to work on analyzing data in a transparent way to quickly address critical questions. Abernethy described this effort as an example of how FDA is increasing its capacity to use these datasets and to work toward better understanding about (1) data that are fit-for-purpose, (2) problems with data characterization and quality, (3) appropriate and accurate analyses, and (4) the integration of new capabilities such as artificial intelligence. Transparency

---

[3] More information about FDA's action to harness real-world data to inform COVID-19 response efforts is available at https://evidenceaccelerator.org (accessed December 17, 2020).

in this process allows everyone to observe and comment on the work being done, she added.

Data Sharing in Regenerative Medicine

Do the low numbers of clinical trials, patients, and products inherent in regenerative medicine make shared databases necessary?, asked Krishnendu Roy. Would FDA, he continued, participate in a registry containing de-identified patient measurements and outcomes that allows for sharing datasets large enough to include characterization measurements and manufacturing parameters? Abernethy noted that other areas of medicine, such as rare diseases, also have low numbers and a similar need to devise sharing mechanisms to allow data aggregation in order to achieve adequate cohort size and detail. Several different sharing mechanisms exist, including data pooling, which is similar to the data warehousing model, and the federated model. Other models use a series of linkage techniques to aggregate data, while an intentional model develops single, core registries or parallel registries that are joined. Different models have value for different types of tasks, so Abernethy suggested that when one selects a model, it is important to consider the tasks that will be initiated and it may be helpful to think of datasets as central resources that can be curated in such a way that one can make comparisons among them. Examples of reference datasets can be found in the laboratory and microbiology space, she said. Abernethy did not comment on the specific direction FDA plans to take in this area, but she suggested that the organization's Orphan Products Grants Program may pertain to this topic.[4]

Does FDA, Plant asked, offer incentives to stimulate data sharing among companies that may have proprietary information concerns? Companies may have different motivations depending on the circumstances, Abernethy said; the specific circumstances involved may lend themselves to one of the four models of data sharing previously mentioned. For instance, with rare diseases the patient community may provide the motivation to create a sharing mechanism. Currently, the COVID-19 pandemic combined with available health technologies have created a business opportunity to establish aggregated pools of data and perform high-level curation in order to sell those data to downstream purchasers. FDA does provide direct stimulation in certain areas, Abernethy said, with the Orphan Products Grants Program being one example.

---

[4]More information about the Orphan Products Grants Program is available at https://www.fda.gov/industry/developing-products-rare-diseases-conditions/orphan-products-grants-program (accessed December 8, 2020).

Technical and Human Capabilities Required for Systems Thinking

Which areas related to systems level thinking warrant attention? Plant asked. Data sharing, data linkage, and having individuals with the abilities required to work with these datasets are critical areas, Abernethy replied. To become adequately equipped to receive this type of work, FDA is currently developing the ability to work with similar datasets and to cross-verify results from different teams, which requires technical capabilities and appropriate expertise.

Given that this work involves both hard systems (e.g., modeling, mathematics) and soft systems, such as human interaction, Plant asked Abernethy what she views as the bigger challenge: getting humans to understand the changes and to work together or getting the mathematical and technical details right. Abernethy reflected on her experiences of earning a Ph.D. in informatics, serving as the founding director of the Center for Learning Health Care at Duke University, and building datasets at a health technology company before coming to FDA. Throughout those experiences, she said, the most challenging aspect of bringing data together and applying them across disparate fields was the human component. This underscores the need to develop a common language to ensure an equal voice for all stakeholders, from mathematicians to clinicians to drug developers.

Impact of Systems Thinking on Cost Reduction

Could systems thinking, a workshop participant asked, contribute to reducing the costs of cell and gene therapy, and, if so, does FDA have a role in achieving that goal? Abernethy noted that cost is not specifically considered in FDA's medical product approval process for safety and effectiveness. However, efficiency does directly influence the overall cost of product development, and systems thinking will likely make trials more efficient, which should in turn affect issues related to cost. Additionally, she said, she expects that systems thinking will likely cause a shift toward platform thinking as it relates to cell and gene therapies, which could create scalable opportunities and thus reduce costs. Systems thinking in health care delivery, especially for therapies such as chimeric antigen receptor (CAR) T cell therapy, can increase optimization across the service chain and have resulting value. Although these types of datasets can increase efficiency, they are expensive to generate and can be costly to manage. She cautioned that a focus on generating and using these datasets as a cost-saving measure can potentially undermine the ability to perform this work with the quality and credibility that is expected.

USING SYSTEMS THINKING APPROACHES FOR CELL THERAPY PRODUCT DEVELOPMENT

Role of Patients in Systems-Based Thinking

Olson described his experience as patient number 2 on the initial University of Pennsylvania clinical trial of CART19.[5] At the time of the clinical trial, the only recipients of the treatment had been mice, so there was little knowledge regarding what to expect in humans. In serving as a patient advocate with CMaT, Olson has followed CAR T therapeutic research and the tremendous variability in patient response and toxicities. He emphasized that patients have an important role to play in providing feedback about their experiences with CAR T therapy in clinical trials. Given that it is an individualized therapy and each patient is different, he said, it will be crucial to be able to predict what patients should expect from the therapy in terms of both experience and outcome. In talking with patients who are considering or beginning CAR T cell therapy, he has found that the most common question he is asked is what they should expect. He gives the same answer as physicians do: that every patient is an individual, and responses can vary. However, Olson said he also tries to include a message of hope. As a patient, he said, he is excited to see systems-based approaches being used to gain a better understanding of an individual patient's biological make-up and of how patients are likely to respond to a therapy because that will be of great value in supporting these patients.

Iterative Process of Defining Critical Quality Attributes

Temple discussed the value of systems thinking to therapeutic cell product development. Cell products are a relatively new and growing area of therapy development. Unlike small molecules, cells are highly complex and dynamic, and cell products are often mixtures of multiple cell types. Because the complexity involved in these products far exceeds that of typical drugs, she suggested distilling down that complexity to the critical quality attributes of each cell product that should be monitored during good manufacturing practices (GMPs).

Temple described three steps in the iterative process of defining critical quality attributes. The first step is to gather key information about the cell product. Cutting-edge techniques, such as high-content image analysis, single-cell gene expression, and protein expression, can be used to acquire a wealth of information about cells. New techniques are also continually

---

[5]More information about clinical trial NCT01029366 is available at https://clinicaltrials.gov/ct2/show/NCT01029366 (accessed December 8, 2020).

being created for cell study. At this step of the process, specific data, methodologies, and time points should be selected strategically to generate in-depth and wide information, Temple said. The next step is to collect information about the patient and his or her response to treatment, including data on genetics, blood analytics, imaging, and functional outcome measures. Collecting these data, which are complex, can be costly to both the patient and the study, so both the types of data and the time-frame for collection should be carefully considered. The third step is to integrate the information and correlate product characteristics with patient outcomes in order to identify critical quality attributes, which are then incorporated into the GMP process. Temple emphasized that this is an iterative process that requires systems-level thinking. Although the challenges involved are considerable, she said, this process of defining critical quality attributes is essential to ensure reliable manufacturing of products that are safe and effective for patients.

Process of Cell Therapy Development as a System

Manian discussed the process of cell therapy development as a system (see Figure 3-1) and explored how systems thinking approaches from the field of engineering can affect manufacturing efficiencies. In any manufacturing process, he said, raw materials—cells, in this case—have a substantial impact on the output of the process. However, in the development of cell therapies, cell procurement often receives inadequate consideration with respect to procurement timing, phenotypic distribution, cell health, and the impact of apheresis on cell quality. The next step in the process after procurement is cell selection and enrichment, which involves considerations of yield and the health of the cells that will later be engineered. Cell activation and stimulation make up the next step, and here the focus is on achieving consistent, repeatable, and well-controlled activation. Adopting a philosophy that the "process is the product"—which often frames the process as a series of steps performed repeatedly in an identical fashion—can lead one to overlook the tremendous degree of interaction among components of the process, Manian said. On the other hand, taking the appropriate measurements during this phase can facilitate adjustments as needed between the components of the process. During the next step—genetic modification (i.e., genetic engineering)—receptor density and epitope conservation are often overlooked, despite the technological capability and ability to observe those variables on the production floor. The next step is cell expansion, in which considerations of quantity and cell health are important. The concentration and purity of the drug product need to be monitored as expanded cells are harvested, he said. During the formulation and release of the drug product, the focus is on function and pyrogenicity as well as on the impact

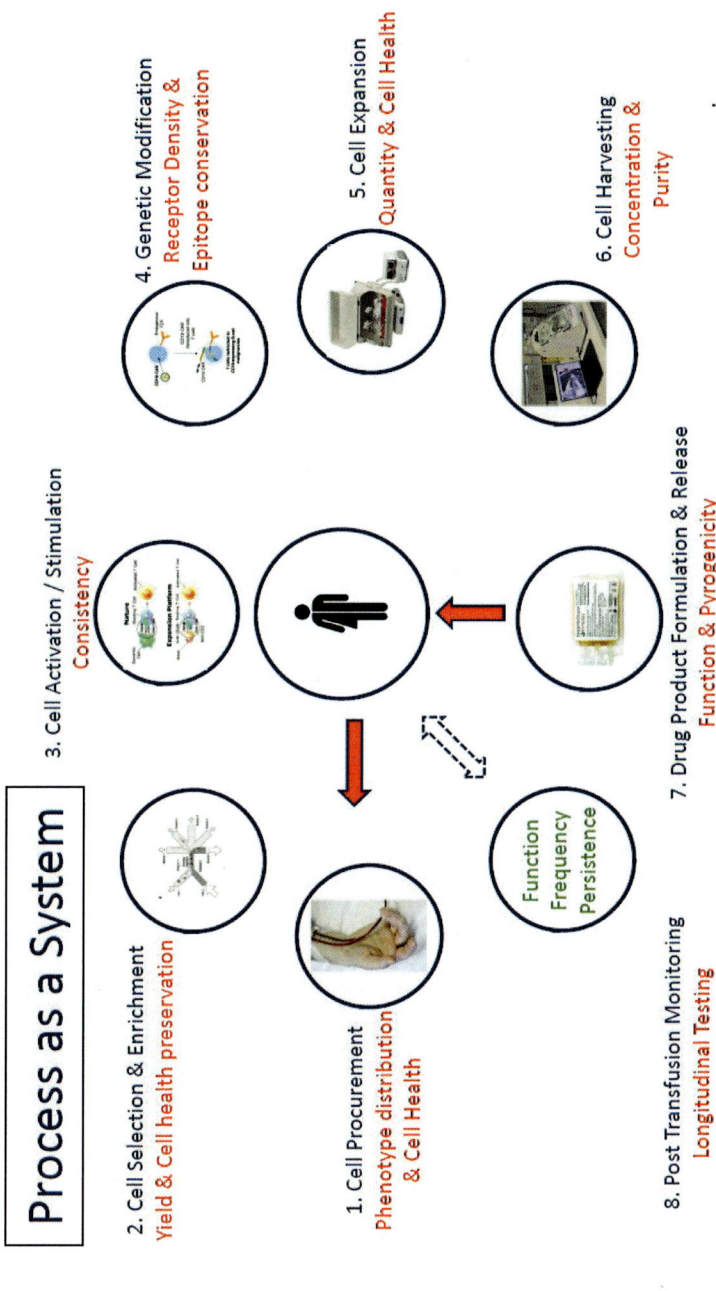

FIGURE 3-1 Process of cell therapy development as a system.
SOURCE: Bala Manian workshop presentation, October 22, 2020.

of pyrogenicity after infusion because cell and gene product raw materials are not sterile. The final step is post-transfusion patient monitoring, which is conducted longitudinally over a long period of time. The data generated throughout all components of this manufacturing system are then collected across patients and used to improve the ability to produce consistent and reliable products. This system can be characterized at the component level by examining the interactions among components. Furthermore, Manian said, this process can be framed as a closed-loop system, which can act as a guidance in the adjustment of parameters to produce a reliable product that is consistent over time.

Systems Biology in Support of Cell Therapy

Bot described how systems biology thinking is used in the context of CAR T cell therapy. He provided an overview of CAR T cell technology and the modern approaches based on machine learning that are used to understand the separate components of the system and bring them together in an integrative model. The current version of CAR T cell therapy involves genetically engineering lymphocytes harvested through apheresis from each individual patient. The critical step in this multi-step manufacturing process is the use of viral vectors to introduce a synthetic gene; this gene expresses a synthetic molecule that enables immune T cells to lock onto target cells, recognize them, and eliminate them from the body. To date, the three products that have been approved in this area are all directed at B-cell lymphomas and leukemias and express an antigen called cluster of differentiation 19, or CD19.

There are data available from both clinical and post-marketing studies on thousands of patients who have been treated with CAR T cells, Bot said. This provides an opportunity to integrate data from manufacturing, delivery, and patient outcomes into larger models, potentially contributing to an unprecedented understanding of how immune cells interact with various organs of the body and how they mediate response or toxicities. To move these efforts forward, Bot said, three questions should be considered:

- How can we better characterize products by identifying the quality product attributes that matter most?
- How can we better define and understand the mechanisms of treatment resistance—either primary treatment resistance or secondary treatment resistance (relapse)—in order to optimize such processes as manufacturing, clinical protocols, and the development of next-generation interventions?

- How can we understand the novel toxicities associated with CAR T cells, which are potent in terms of immunological activity and can lead to toxicities (e.g., cytokine release syndrome)?

All of the information collected can be fed back into biostatistics databases and used to generate models through collaboration among those with expertise in multiple disciplines, Bot said. The components of these models (e.g., product attributes, tumor characteristics, clinical outcomes, pharmacokinetics, pharmacodynamics) can then be interrogated and combined. Next, machine learning is used to define and prioritize the components that have the most influence on the outcome and which components can be used as leads for process optimization, next-generation interventions, and product characterization.

This process and its component parts constitute a systems biology approach, Bot said. He presented a model of CAR T cell therapy that depicts how CAR T cells work, why they sometimes fail, and how they are identified. The critical product attributes of CAR T cells include intrinsic T cell fitness or expansion capability, T cell polyfunctionality, CAR functional avidity, and receptor density. These attributes influence the outcome of therapy. Additionally, the model incorporates tumor-associated factors and other patient characteristics that interact with product attributes, producing information on pharmacokinetics, pharmacodynamics profiles, clinical efficacy, and toxicity. Tumor biology research is rapidly expanding the knowledge base about the role of the tumor immune microenvironment and of how the oncogenic landscape interacts with product attributes to influence clinical response or treatment resistance. This knowledge helps optimize the manufacturing process and maximize the number of specialized T cells that mediate clinical efficacy without increasing the toxicity profile. In parallel, systems biology thinking enables the creation of networks of cells and molecules that jointly determine the outcome of T cell interventions, including inflammatory toxicities. Bot said that this type of thinking helps narrow down molecules and actionable targets involved in managing, mitigating, and preventing toxicities associated with CAR T cell interventions.

DISCUSSION

Implementing Systems-Based Thinking in Cell Characterization

Throughout the session, Lebkowski said, the importance of identifying cell types, cell function, cell phenotype, and cell properties was demonstrated. How, she asked, could systems-based thinking be implemented in, for example, the process of cell characterization? The type of data gathering for a cell product that Temple described in her presentation is not particularly compatible with a GMP process, she said. Rather, it is used to understand the product in depth in a research environment. For example, this type of high-level data analysis of a product is used to look at gene expression at the single-cell level and to identify the emergent properties that pertain to pathways and cell states. Multimodal integration may involve sets of omics data (e.g., single-cell transcriptomics), live-cell imaging, and computer-based imaging. Bringing together different modalities to make sense of this information is challenging, but these large-scale analyses can be used to identify emergent properties and predict how to develop products that are safe and useful. Then the product needs to be investigated thoroughly in a research setting to determine how to integrate the different forms of data in order to select which product should be put through a GMP process, she said.

Lebkowski asked whether Temple envisions a focus on critical quality attributes—perhaps tweaking or revising them as part of the product development process—to better understand the function and the interaction of particular cells in a human. To do so, Temple said, patient data will need to be gathered and compared with what is being discovered about the cell product. This is challenging because (1) it is demanding from the patients' perspective, (2) it is expensive to study in a clinical trial, and (3) it can be difficult to determine what to measure and for how long to measure it. However, critical quality attributes cannot be identified until patient data, including data about response, are incorporated into these analyses, Temple said.

Implementing Systems-Based Approaches in CAR T Cell Therapy

A major challenge in implementing systems-based approaches in CAR T cell therapy, Bot said, is the need to scale up and scale out the datasets in the post-commercial setting. He and his colleagues are trying to harmonize biomarker approaches and protocols by partnering with registries such as the international or regional bone marrow transplant registries and are working with physicians and patients to obtain appropriate consent for additional data collection. It is, Bot said, "absolutely critical" to identify, train, and validate predictive algorithms for CAR T cell intervention toxicities and efficacy. There has been significant progress over the past 5 years in terms of knowledge about the key determinants of response to CAR T cell intervention. However, he said, more work is needed to create strong predictive algorithms based on systems biology thinking, which can only be accomplished in partnership with appropriate stakeholders in the commercial post-marketing setting. To forge such relationships, he has partnered with academic collaborators and other major comprehensive cancer centers that are collecting data. Through collaboration, he said, data can be deposited and analyzed in an organized fashion.

Integrating Systems-Based Approaches into Manufacturing

What, Lebowski asked, are some of the opportunities and challenges in integrating systems-based approaches into the manufacturing system? Manian pointed to the intersection between design thinking and systems thinking. Design thinking is often involved in development in considering how a product will be manufactured. Although the measurement technologies used to understand and establish mechanisms of cell therapy are complex, generational biomarkers or surrogate measurements can provide insights into these mechanisms. Manian suggested that measurements of system components should not be used to understand a process, but instead should be implemented on the manufacturing floor. Because manufacturing is a continuous process that cannot be stopped for lengthy periods of time, measurements in a manufacturing space must be conducted within 15 minutes or so and must provide information in a way that is actionable. Viewed in that context, there are many tools that are currently available to take measurements at each component of the process, Manian said. Based on the information gathered, adjustments can be made in the subsequent process in response to the indications of the data. This need not be an open loop system; it can also be a closed-loop system. He suggested that information on the incoming material is the point at which interaction currently needs to occur because little characterization is currently being done in this area. Moving the process to the point of cell procurement can have a huge impact on the overall control of the processes, he added. Furthermore, each component of a system can be framed in terms of making measurements. For example, viral vectors are currently examined only in terms of control-arm viral vector delivery. However, many other components can be explored, such as generated receptor densities, uniformity, variation across patients, impact on cell health, and the survivability of engineered cells. Manian suggested that, over time, the processes of characterizations will lead to a better understanding of the overall manufacturing process. "Just as we understand interaction between cells, we need to understand the interaction between components of the manufacturing system," he said.

Improving Patient Data Collection

Given the variability driven by different starting materials and diverse patient characteristics, Lebkowski asked, are clinical trials collecting sufficient data about patients and products to integrate aspects of manufacturing or patient variability into systems-based thinking? If it is not sufficient, she continued, which types of data should be collected and how can data collection, particularly from patients, be improved? Bot replied that CAR T cells are based on the patient's own immune system, which is a collection of heterogeneous T cells, B cells, and other immune cells, and in this case the T cells are of particular interest. Although patient heterogeneity in T cells is overwhelming, collecting data about that heterogeneity will be critical for identifying the most important attributes in patients' pre-treatment immune systems in terms of influencing product characteristics and subsequent clinical outcomes. In the face of this heterogeneity, fully leveraging this opportunity will require single-cell omics analysis of characteristics such as T cell fitness, expansion capability, resistance to apoptosis (i.e., cell death), and the ability to engage multiple immune programs simultaneously, which seems to be linked to clinical performance. All of this information can be used to build better predictive algorithms that are more actionable in delivery, Bot said, because they rely on data from pre-manufacturing characteristics of the immune system. Furthermore, this will help pave the way to a new generation of cell interventions based on designer, off-the-shelf cells that are sourced either from stem cells differentiated ex vivo or from well-defined donors. This would result in a tremendous reduction in inter-patient variability in the next-generation products, he said.

Could the collection of induced pluripotent stem (iPS) cells from individual patients help, Lebkowski asked, to tease out some degree of heterogeneity from patient to patient? That is an interesting idea, Temple said, because iPS cell technology is enhancing the ability to produce many different types of tissue. This tissue can be produced in three dimensions to build organoids that are representative of gut, brain, skin, and inner ear. iPS cells could be used to study individuals, although CAR T technology may not yet have advanced far enough to create the relevant cells. Temple said that a challenge with iPS cells is their tendency to be in an immature state, but work is under way to learn how to mature those cells.

"We look for a lost key under the light because that is where the light is," Manian said. Typically, cell therapy is approached in terms of making measurements with existing instrumentation; instead, he said, the process should start with defining the parameters critical to quality in order to determine the type of measurements needed. New methods developed to generate information about phenomena—such as cytokine profiling and phenotyping—across multiple patients and multiple types of drugs for the same disease state will likely further reveal how systems biology can affect manufacturing.

Are there opportunities, Lebkowski asked, to improve patient communication, for example, by explaining why organizations and developers of regenerative medicine therapies are trying to collect extensive panels of data from subjects who might be entering a trial? Olson said he has found from both his own personal experience and from his advocacy work engaging with patients contemplating this therapy that a major challenge is to distill the large amount of data that already exist and to find ways to apply those data to each individual patient and predict what patients can expect based on their individual characteristics. Information already available should be framed more effectively for patients considering or beginning CAR T cell therapy so as to help them understand the therapy. The huge growth in the volume of CAR T data over the past decade is astounding, he added, but continuing to collect data on each individual's experience and matching it to biological parameters is the work that still lies ahead.

Approaching Systems Thinking via Collaboration

Given the substantial resources required for systems thinking approaches, Lebkowski asked if a single sponsor would be adequate or if a consortium would be required. Kite Pharma, Inc., began this work, Bot said, by launching a consortium with large academic organizations that participate in clinical trials and sponsor research at the post-marketing stage for both axicabtagene ciloleucel (brand name Yescarta®) and brexucabtagene autoleucel (brand name Tecartus®), the two Kite products approved to date. Current work involves generating big data, using a harmonized biomarker protocol aligned with a schedule of assessments, integrating data via methodologies and analytics aligned with a single command structure, and analyzing data with pre-specified protocols and machine learning. However, advancing the field by accelerating real-world data generation will require a consortium across different sponsors and organizations in the industry to share data and collaborate with regulators. Bot suggested that this would contribute to optimizing patient management by learning how to increase the rate of durable responses and predicting or mitigating toxicities that may require intensive management in a hospital setting.

Costs of Not Implementing Systems Thinking

What are the costs to the field of regenerative medicine, Lebkowski asked, if systems thinking approaches are not implemented? Temple described a real-world example of a company that was generating a cell therapy for spinal cord injury and discovered that some element of the manufacturing process led to failure of that product. Although the product may have passed the criteria for release, it was clear that important aspects of the product were not being captured in the data collected. The clinical process for GMP is expensive because of the complexity of cells, she added. In her experience, she said, more comprehensive testing before release would be ideal, but it becomes cost prohibitive. However, an inadequate understanding of all of components in a system also comes at a cost (i.e., the cost of failure of the enterprise and, most importantly, of failure to deliver a beneficial product to patients). Temple underscored the need to characterize therapeutic products more carefully and to integrate that information with patient data to predict responses more accurately and identify subpopulations of patients that are most likely to benefit from those products.

Manian highlighted the need to standardize processes to establish a framework with competencies that can be implemented. If systems thinking is not applied, then individualized patient-by-patient processes will remain unaffordable for a large segment of the population. Bot added that the costs of not implementing systems thinking are the missed opportunities to expand the footprint of potentially curative interventions in early disease stages and to benefit as many patients as possible.

4

Challenges Associated with Data Collection, Aggregation, and Sharing

---

Important Points Highlighted by Individual Speakers

- The transition toward open science in omics analysis and disease modeling can be supported by encouraging the team-based production of knowledge (e.g., via consortia) and by incentivizing collaboration through competitions and challenges. (Omberg)
- Model-to-data challenges can catalyze crowdsourced innovations without compromising the confidentiality of patients' biomedical data. (Omberg)
- Pooling and harmonizing real-world clinical data collected across a large, distributed health system into a large-scale, centralized database can facilitate the clinical stratification of patients, expedite large trials, enable comparative effectiveness studies, and realize cost savings across the system. (Butte)
- Real-world patient-related data have many uses beyond product development and regulation; ultimately, these data should be used to communicate with and support patients receiving novel types of therapeutics. (Butte)
- In the field of regenerative medicine, the amount of data collected will never be sufficient to fully capture all of a product's critical quality attributes; thus, researchers should focus on ways to leverage the data that are currently available. (Butte, Omberg)
- The use of interoperable standards for electronic health records can facilitate data sharing and contribute to developing a lingua franca across industry, academia, and regulators. (Butte, Omberg)

The third session of the workshop, moderated by Sadik Kassim of Vor Biopharma, explored challenges associated with data collection, aggregation, and sharing. The session featured presentations on how open science can be applied in omics and disease modeling and also on the use of big data in clinically stratifying patients. This session's objectives were to discuss how big data can be used to identify which patients will respond best to a particular regenerative medicine and to highlight challenges in data collection and data sharing such as small sample sizes in clinical trials, proprietary issues, and patient privacy.

TOWARD OPEN SCIENCE IN OMICS ANALYSIS AND DISEASE MODELING

Larsson Omberg, the vice president of systems biology at Sage Bionetworks, spoke about the opportunities and challenges involved in using open science approaches in omics analyses and disease modeling. Sage Bionetworks, helps research communities develop reliable outcomes to advance the understanding of human health by harnessing the power of open and collaborative science. He added, however, that open science should be supported with appropriate incentives and structures to catalyze innovation.

Shift Toward Team-Based Production of Knowledge in Biomedical Research

In recent years teams have come to increasingly dominate the production of knowledge in the field of biomedical research (Wuchty et al., 2007), although the biological sciences have lagged behind other hard sciences, such as physics and astronomy, in shifting toward this type of team-based production of knowledge. This shift has been driven largely by the increasing costs associated with cutting-edge research, Omberg said. The fields of physics and astronomy made this shift to large-scale collaborative efforts and team-based production of knowledge earlier than biomedical research, where it emerged in the 2000s. In the field of genomics, this transition was also spurred by the large costs associated with data production. Historically, those costs were related to the expensive technologies that were required, but now the costs result primarily from the large sample sizes needed to conduct research. Furthermore, researchers have found that in the fields of science and technology, large teams tend to develop, while small teams are more likely to disrupt (Wu et al., 2019). Sage Bionetworks works mainly with large teams by helping and enabling large consortia, but there have been cases of disruption when individuals within teams have brought new ideas to bear, he added.

Moving Toward Open Science

Omberg said he prefers the term "open science" over "open data" because open data represent just one component of many in open science which should all be considered together. The volume of open data has increased substantially since 2004, as demonstrated by the growing rate of Internet searches for the term "open data" and related concepts over the past decade. Underlying concepts of fairness and accessibility are particularly strong drivers of many open research efforts. The U.S. government also has a strong interest in open data, he added. For example, the National Institutes of Health (NIH) introduced a genomics data sharing policy in 2014[1] that requires all data to be made open within 6 months after generation. Scientists are sometimes reluctant to use open methods due to a lack of incentives for collaborating and sharing data, Omberg said, however this attitude is changing, particularly among younger researchers. Making science open is a good first step, he continued, but it is not enough: incentives must be adjusted appropriately (Chen et al., 2019). In physics research, for example, large numbers of astronomical datasets were made available openly, yet much of the data went unused. Incentive structures may help to ensure that scientists work with data that are made available, he said.

Consortium-Based Collaboration in Alzheimer's Disease Research

Sage Bionetworks is involved in numerous collaborative projects and consortia, primarily in the fields of cancer research, neurodegeneration, and neuropsychiatric disease, Omberg said. As an example of collaborative science, he described the Accelerating Medicines Partnership Alzheimer's Disease (AMP AD).[2] This public–private consortium was established to bring together NIH, biopharmaceutical and life sciences companies, and nonprofit organizations to develop new diagnostics and treatments and address the lack of biological targets for Alzheimer's disease (AD). Although AD has been cured in mice, not a single clinical trial has succeeded in curing the disease in humans despite investments of billions of dollars from both pharmaceutical companies and governments (Franco and Cedazo-Minguez, 2014). Research on AD has traditionally been focused on a limited set of targets, so the AMP AD was established to expand the number of AD targets by using systems biology approaches. Sage Bionetworks has taken on a coordinating role to facilitate numerous additional related efforts, including

---

[1] For more information on the NIH genomics data sharing policy, see https://osp.od.nih.gov/scientific-sharing/genomic-data-sharing (accessed January 19, 2021).

[2] More information about the Accelerating Medicines Partnership is available at https://fnih.org/what-we-do/programs/amp (accessed November 30, 2020).

- MODEL-AD,[3] which is developing mice models of AD;
- Resilience-AD,[4] which is studying the resilience of AD;
- M^{2}OVE-AD,[5] which studies vascularization;
- Psych-AD,[6] which studies the interaction between neuropsychiatric disease and AD; and
- TREAT-AD,[7] which is working to develop target-enabling packages to help with the preclinical development of drugs using targets identified through AMP AD.

At Sage, there is a data repository containing more than 17,000 biosamples and 15 genomic data types from 7,261 human donors collected from a range of sources, Omberg said. These open-access data are used to build algorithms (e.g., RNA-seq processing, proteomic analysis, single-cell RNA) to generate analytical results that can be used to identify new targets for AD.

Making genomic data useful across studies requires substantial collaborative work, Omberg emphasized. To illustrate, he described how RNA-seq analysis[8] is conducted collaboratively within the AMP AD consortium. Initially, the consortium was working with highly heterogeneous data from postmortem brain samples collected using varying technologies and analytical approaches, which made it impossible to make direct comparisons. To homogenize these data, several groups within the consortium worked together to create a canonical dataset that could be used in downstream analysis to derive insights. This type of data pooling allows different groups to conduct their own analyses on the same dataset, he added. A working group was formed to evaluate the methods used by different teams for these analyses, as well as some pre-published methodologies, in order to begin consensus modeling across these methods using a multimethod co-expression network analysis and differential expression meta-analysis. A consensus was established by developing a common set of outputs generated by those methods. This was used to identify a canonical set of existing

---

[3]More information about MODEL-AD is available at https://sagebionetworks.org/research-projects/model-ad (accessed December 22, 2020).

[4]More information about Resilience-AD is available at https://grants.nih.gov/grants/guide/rfa-files/RFA-AG-17-061.html (accessed December 22, 2020).

[5]More information about M^{2}OVE-AD is available at https://adknowledgeportal.synapse.org/Explore/Programs/DetailsPage?Program=M2OVE-AD (accessed December 22, 2020).

[6]More information about Psych-AD is available at https://grants.nih.gov/grants/guide/rfa-files/RFA-MH-19-510.html (accessed December 22, 2020).

[7]More information about TREAT-AD is available at https://sagebionetworks.org/research-projects/treat-ad (accessed December 22, 2020).

[8]More information about RNA sequencing analysis is available at https://www.ncbi.nlm.nih.gov/pmc/articles/PMC6096346 (accessed January 16, 2021).

networks; comparative module analysis was used to identify differences (Wan et al., 2020).

These analyses revealed a sizable degree of overlap between these groups' work, Omberg said. A large subset of these consensus networks contained items that were found commonly across many methodologies, but did not correspond to known AD biology, thus highlighting the large universe of unknown or poorly understood AD biology. Described by Omberg as "the dark matter of AD biology," these unknowns are of great interest in the context of identifying new possible targets and sources of disease. However, he said, much more research will be needed to operationalize this insight in a useful way (e.g., by using these newly identified targets in drug development). To that end, NIH's National Institute on Aging has invested in TREAT-AD. The aim is to develop target-enabling packages for targets identified through the AMP AD consortium, to help identify which may be "druggable," and to develop tools that can be used by those who work on drug development. This often involves expanding targets into a large set of possible targets based on "druggability," then using associated targets through network models.

Incentivizing Collaboration Through Competitions and Crowdsourcing

Omberg presented an example of a collaboration that brings working groups together to crowdsource solutions to fundamental biomedical questions: Dialogue on Reverse Engineering Assessment and Methods (DREAM) Challenges.[9] When a new method is developed, its developer often tests and validates the method themselves, he said, which can result in better-than-average findings. DREAM Challenges were created to separate development from benchmarking and to address problems related to "self-assessment," which has impeded the translation and dissemination of biomedical tools and methods. New incentives would help to push research communities to develop domain standards and benchmarks, he suggested. By posing these challenges as an open problem, this project is intended to quickly explore a larger space of solutions that can be generated through crowd sourcing.

mPower is a series of mobile research studies aimed at understanding the progression of Parkinson's disease (PD) in individuals, Omberg said.[10] In one of those studies, the researchers recruited individuals with PD to

---

[9]More information about the DREAM Challenges program is available at http://dreamchallenges.org (accessed December 11, 2020).

[10]More information about mPower is available at https://sagebionetworks.org/research-projects/mpower-researcher-portal (accessed December 11, 2020).

measure their symptoms using accelerometers and on-screen interactions via smartphones (Bot et al., 2016). In accordance with Sage Bionetworks's values, this study released its first 6 months of data upon compilation and before analysis, making it a public resource.[11] Within the first year, more than 130 individuals from 35 different institutions had requested access to the data, which eventually led to more than a dozen publications. However, several of these publications arrived at insights about these data that were inaccurate, Omberg said. He attributed this, in part, to the fact that some of those who accessed the data were better versed in machine learning than in disease. Thus, they did not consider the covariates and noise characteristics in the data that might affect the disease or measurements.

Competitions can help incentivize innovation, Omberg said. He described a challenge that Sage Bionetworks held to help develop impartial benchmarks from mPower data. Sage Bionetworks asked researchers to build diagnostic digital biomarkers using the mPower accelerometer data to determine if an individual has PD and, if so, the severity of the individual's disease. Previous analyses of these accelerometer and digital wearable data conducted by a group of experts had taken years to develop a diagnostic biomarker which had an area under the curve (AUC) of 0.69, which is not a good level of predictive accuracy. Through the challenge, more than 300 groups accessed the data and used them to build their own models; within weeks, the winning group had built a measure with an AUC of 0.84, far exceeding the predictive accuracy of the one developed by the expert group (Sieberts et al., 2021). This new measure led to a 20 percent increase in performance. This was a prime example of how incentivizing competition can create better quality work. Importantly, this entire effort was made open source so that the data, tools, and collaborative methodologies can be reused.[12]

Challenges Related to Data Governance

Many of the data needed to answer important clinical questions are not open data, Omberg said. Ethical considerations as well as regulatory considerations such as the Health Insurance Portability and Accountability Act (HIPAA) in the United States and General Data Protection Regulation 2016/679 in Europe restrict the access and use of data. These considerations are rooted in data governance: the freedoms, constraints, and incentives that determine how two or more parties manage—among themselves and

---

[11] More information about the mPower Researcher Community is available at https://www.synapse.org/#!Synapse:syn4993293/wiki/247859 (accessed December 1, 2020).

[12] Sage Bionetworks's open-source tools are available at https://github.com/Sage-Bionetworks/mhealthtools (accessed December 1, 2020).

with others—the ingress, storage, analysis, and egress of data tools, methods, and knowledge. Because data governance involves two or more parties, there are often associated issues related to communication, negotiation, and interpersonal power dynamics, Omberg said. Data governance also affects software, storage, computer power, and know-how while access to external digital resources will also be involved. Data governance structures and their attributes can be characterized in terms of their associated freedoms and availability, Omberg said. The most closed and restricted data would rank lowest in both freedoms and availability, while data from open sources and citizen science have high degrees of freedom and availability.

Model-to-Data Challenge in Digital Mammography

One such option for governance that Sage Bionetworks has experimented with is model-to-data challenges, Omberg said, which provide an opportunity to spur innovation without compromising the confidentiality of biomedical data (Guinney and Saez-Rodriguez, 2018). These challenges are appropriate for addressing specific research questions rather than general purpose analysis, Omberg noted. Challenge participants submit containerized models, built using training data, to a privacy-conserving cloud platform. Model submissions are then validated using datasets containing patient-identifying information that are not available to the challenge participants in order to develop competition leaderboards and benchmarks. For example, the Digital Mammography DREAM Challenge[13] was a model-to-data challenge where challenge participants built models to predict whether mammogram images contained breast cancer. It included data collected from 86,801 women in 146,201 digital mammography examinations conducted at Kaiser Permanente; 1,006 of these exams were cancer-positive. A total of 640,394 images were collected, along with clinical and demographic information. Dozens of teams participated by submitting models based on deep-learning methods which were trained and validated on these images without the participants ever having seen or accessed the data directly.

USING BIG DATA FOR CLINICAL STRATIFICATION OF PATIENTS

Atul Butte, the Priscilla Chan and Mark Zuckerberg Distinguished Professor and the director of the Bakar Computational Health Sciences

---

[13]More information about the Digital Mammography DREAM Challenge is available at https://sagebionetworks.org/research-projects/digital-mammography-dream-challenge (accessed December 11, 2020).

Institute at the University of California, San Francisco, discussed how big data can be used for the clinical stratification of patients. He opened with an overview that emphasized the size and complexity of the University of California Health (UCH) system. The system comprises ten campuses and three national labs, with approximately 200,000 employees and about 250,000 students per year, Butte said, and its health system includes 20 health professional schools, and the UCH system trains half of all the medical students and residents in California. Around 5,000 faculty physicians and 12,000 nurses work in the UCH system, with 100,000 outside doctors writing orders on patients within the system. The UCH system also includes five National Cancer Institute (NCI) comprehensive cancer centers. The system has a policy of institutional review board reliance, whereby approvals in one campus can easily be applied in other campuses, and it also benefits from centralized contracting.

In 2016 the UCH system and UnitedHealth Group entered into an agreement to form a single accountable care organization (ACO) for the entire University of California (UC) system as part of a 10-year strategic relationship with Optum to expand the use of its clinically integrated network services and advanced data analytics services.[14] By their nature, ACOs take on risk; they are paid per member, per month, and must absorb the current prices for delivering care. Moving forward, the UCH system has to determine how it would best practice medicine in order to operate with a single ACO, because the various UC campuses deliver care in different ways. Thus, Butte said, the operational need to harmonize practice data across the entire system motivated the decision to aggregate all of their health data in a single place.

Centralizing Health Care Data Across the University of California Health System

Today, health care data from across the six UC medical schools[15] is stored both locally and in the centralized UCH data warehouse.[16] These data include basic data from more than 15 million patients treated since 2005 and detailed electronic health record (EHR) data on more than 7 million patients since EHR systems were installed in early 2012, providing the

---

[14] More information about UHC's ACO is available at https://hitconsultant.net/2016/10/03/uchealth-united-healthcare-form-new-aco (accessed December 1, 2020).

[15] The six schools are the University of California, San Francisco; University of California, Los Angeles; University of California, Irvine; University of California, Davis; University of California, San Diego; and University of California, Riverside.

[16] Before the coronavirus disease 2019 (COVID-19) pandemic, data backups were scheduled monthly, according to Butte; during the COVID-19 pandemic, data backups have been scheduled nightly from midnight to 6:00 a.m. Pacific time.

UCH system with a unique view of its medical system. No other example of comprehensive bulk data sharing across multiple academic medical centers exists in the United States, Butte said. All of the UC medical schools now use Epic for their EHRs, but the central database was built using Observational Medical Outcomes Partnership (OMOP) for the data backend rather than Epic because OMOP is an open vendor-neutral method for storing patient data. Each campus moves its data to OMOP to facilitate centralization using commonly shared and governed tools. As of this writing, the database contains structured data from 2012 to the present, including data for 7.3 million patients, 192 million encounters, 553 million procedures, 739 million medical orders, 661 million diagnosis codes, and 2.1 billion laboratory tests and vital signs. This database includes "everything from Tylenol to chimeric antigen receptor T cells" as well as regulatory data related to California's Office of Statewide Health Planning and Development, pathology and radiology text elements, and California state death index data.[17] Claims data from the UCH system's self-funded plans are also included. Elements of this data system are continuously being harmonized and, with new medications and cellular therapies approved on a weekly to monthly basis, the database must be constantly updated to include the latest terminologies. Data governance policies have been put in place, Butte said, to ensure the safe and respectful use of these data, both internally and externally.

The creation of the UCH system data warehouse has facilitated a range of benefits and improvements, Butte said. Many operational teams within the UCH system now use and benefit from the UCH system data warehouse, which is already saving UC millions of dollars. The UCH system data warehouse has also facilitated the central management of primary care patients. Central tools have been developed to improve the quality of care. For UCH system self-funded health plans, managing costs have led to some decreases in expenses, especially in pharmacy spending. Many UCH system and UC employees participate in the self-funded plans, choosing to receive care from their employer. Thus, there is an alignment of incentives for all parties to ensure that the self-funded plans provide the best possible care to the employees and families within these systems, Butte noted. Some measures can be taken to realize cost savings, including the use of generic medications instead of branded versions. Making a case for data agglomeration and harmonization on the basis of improving research alone can be challenging, Butte said, however, making a compelling business case can

---

[17] Butte explained that in the United States each state must track in-state deaths in order to manage Social Security and other programs. UCH has been contracted to manage these death indices and has merged that data with its central data warehouse.

bring heightened interest to these efforts and attract health system funding to pay for them.

University of California Cancer Consortium

In 2017 the UCH system announced that its five NCI-designated comprehensive cancer centers would collaborate through the newly created University of California Cancer Consortium to help patients benefit from therapies that are only deployed through trials.[18] In 2019 the UCH system saw more than 160,000 cancer patients, a patient volume that Butte estimated to be three to four times the volume at the largest cancer centers in the United States. These types of consortia strengthen the work of smaller individual cancer centers, which benefit from scale through collaboration, Butte said. He presented the University of California Cancer Consortium's Foundation Medicine cancer genomic reports as an example of how the group constructs and represents the entire UC system even with the latest tools used in precision medicine.

The consortium benefits from common contracting and the institutional review board reliance process, allowing the group to scale large trials for cancer and cancer therapies quickly, Butte said. For example, Foundation Medicine performs cancer genomics testing for cancer patients across UC and other institutions. UC can show those gene mutation results along with patient race, ethnicity, age, smoking status, and gender. Furthermore, the consortium is able to collect Foundation Medicine cancer genomics data from across the UCH system in one central database. Butte presented data from the San Francisco, Los Angeles, Irvine, and Davis campuses that showed that *TP53* is the mutated gene most frequently found in UCH system cancer patients who have their cancer sequenced. The consortium can use these data on all genetic mutations, downstream therapies, and cancer cases within this centralized database. The consortium also collects information on the cost and charge data for the drugs used across the UCH system, providing the ability to respond to questions in ways that are similar to—and in some ways enhanced—versus how they are answered by groups such as the Patient-Centered Outcomes Research Institute (PCORI). As an example, Butte described how his team analyzed the system's data on the top 10 drug charges across UCH and found that most of the drugs used are biologics and that drug charges across the UCH system total $1.6 billion. Given that the types of biologics used throughout the UCH system

---

[18] More information about the University of California Cancer Consortium is available at https://www.ucsf.edu/news/2017/09/408271/university-california-cancer-consortium-takes-californias-14-billion-killer (accessed December 1, 2020).

vary, these real-world data enable comparative effectiveness studies to be conducted in order to evaluate these different therapies.

Using Real-World Data from the Cancer Consortium

Another advantage of the UCH system database, Butte said, is that a single researcher can conduct multicenter, real-world evidence studies about the use of a drug. He described preliminary work conducted by a graduate student, Michelle Wang, on the therapeutic axicabtagene ciloleucel (axicel/Yescarta). Across the UCH system, 120 patients have already been treated with this cellular therapy, primarily at the Los Angeles, San Diego, and San Francisco campuses. Wang used the data from the patients treated with the drug within the UCH system and analyzed the patients by race, age, ethnicity, and gender (Neelapu et al., 2017). Wang is now evaluating whether the UCH patients would have qualified for the ZUMA-1 clinical trial for axicabtagene ciloleucel,[19] in which 111 individuals were treated with the study drug. The data available through the consortium can already provide a larger sample than the original trial, Butte said. Wang found that more than half of the UCH patients might not have qualified for the ZUMA-1 trial for a number of potential reasons, including (1) the UCH patients might have had worse health status (e.g., they were on oxygen) during the initial acquisition of cells; (2) their laboratory tests were otherwise abnormal; or (3) they required bridging therapy. The amount of time spent from acquiring the cells to delivering the cells (i.e., "vein-to-vein time") determined eligibility for the trial, Butte said. In the real world this time span is longer than it is in the trial data—especially if patients need bridging therapy—thus precluding their qualification for ZUMA-1. This work highlights the importance of real-world evidence, because patients receiving treatments in the real-world setting may not match the patients studied in randomized controlled trials. Both randomized controlled trials and analysis of real-world patients are valuable, Butte said, but this combination of data will be especially useful in studying regenerative medicines.

Wang also prepared data, largely using automated tools provided by the consortium, which compared progression-free survival and overall survival at 12 months for patients treated with axicabtagene ciloleucel. These rates were comparable to the ZUMA-1 trial, Butte said. The availability of these data allows the UCH system to evaluate why outcomes may vary across UC campuses. Using the consortium's data tools, Wang was able to analyze the number and type of adverse events across individual patients, with a focus on mild and severe neutropenia. She can also build computational tools to extract data from laboratory results, including various

---

[19] See https://clinicaltrials.gov/ct2/show/NCT02348216 (accessed February 10, 2021).

markers and even text notes that can be parsed and used. In addition, Wang has begun working to compare data related to cytokine release syndrome (CRS) and neurotoxicity. These data can be plotted according to multiple grading strategies, and when that was done it revealed that the timeline for CRS varies from the timeline of neurotoxicity and achieves an earlier peak than the neurological symptoms seen in neurotoxicity.

Use Cases for Real-World Data

The UCH system now captures real-world data on all activities within its campuses in its clinical data repositories. "Everything we do and measure on patients is captured now, and the electronic health record is now the legal record for the patient," Butte said. Data should serve more than just academic interests, he emphasized. For example, broad and reliable data can be used to create a strong business case for a specific drug or intervention, which tends to speed up implementation. To enumerate the many potential uses of data—including EHR data, clinical data, and patient-reported data—Butte and his colleague compiled 21 use cases for real-world data (Rudrapatna and Butte, 2020) (see Table 4-1). These uses for real-world data extend far beyond the Food and Drug Administration's requirements for pharmaceutical and biotech companies. Ultimately, Butte said, data should be used to communicate with patients about how they may benefit from treatment, how difficult their treatment will be, and the advantages and disadvantages of various potential therapies they may receive.

DISCUSSION

Establishing a Lingua Franca of Data

In order to promote data sharing, there is a need for a lingua franca, or common language, among industry, regulators, and academia, said session moderator Sadik Kassim. Such a system was established within UCH, but he asked how a lingua franca might be established more broadly. Various standards have been developed, Butte said, including Fast Healthcare Interoperability Resources (FHIR), a federal standard for data formats and an application programming interface for exchanging electronic health records. The UCH system uses this standard primarily to export data to patients via the FHIR feed. Many patients receive these feeds using their smartphone, but FHIR feeds can also be used with other tools and technology devices. For sharing data within health systems, UCH uses OMOP, which is also used by PCORI. OMOP is open source and vendor neutral, Butte said, making it as close as possible to a lingua franca. FHIR and

TABLE 4-1 Use Cases for Real-World Data

Category of Use	Use Cases for Real-World Data
Post-approval safety	• Updating side effect rates • Discovering novel side effects
Supporting regulatory approval	• Conducting single-arm experimental trials • Supporting "digital approvals" • Evaluating biosimilar development
Informing clinical trials design	• Improving patient selection • Increasing efficiency of data collection ("trimming the trials")
Continually establishing efficacy	• Assessing the efficacy–effectiveness gap • Searching for efficacy in specific populations • Informing effect modifiers and precision medicine • Evaluating long-term, post-trial outcomes
Comparative effectiveness	• Integrating costs with comparative effectiveness • Understanding effects of pharmacy practices on health care use • Studying novel on-label pharmaceuticals versus older off-label drugs
Studying the practice of medicine	• Improving quality of practice and reducing medical errors • Standardizing care and care delivery • Studying the effect of payors on medical care • Evaluating impact of new-generation diagnostics on outcomes
Data-driven decision support	• Improving clinical decision support: the provider perspective • Improving clinical decision support: the patient perspective • Improving clinical decision support: the community perspective

SOURCES: Atul Butte workshop presentation, October 22, 2020. Adapted from Rudrapatna and Butte, 2020.

OMOP both refer to other standards, so they do not eliminate the need to keep track of vocabularies and the names of pharmaceuticals. The FHIR and OMOP are used far less commonly in the field of digital health, Omberg said. The lack of consistent standards has caused some difficulty in Omberg's work, especially in working across datasets. Acknowledging the positive impact of the use of FHIR for medical records affirmed the importance of developing standards, he said.

Expanding to a National Data-Sharing System

A member of the audience asked whether any efforts are under way to expand the system described by Butte beyond California and how the field of regenerative medicine can use the type of data centralization implemented in the UCH system. There are no immediate plans for expansion outside of California, Butte said, although there are some decentralized national efforts, such as PCORI and private efforts such as TriNetX.[20] A business case would have to be presented to motivate the creation of a national centralized database, he said, but such a case may be difficult to make. To highlight this challenge, he asked why stakeholders would choose to share data for reasons other than getting grants and publishing papers. Kassim agreed that this is a matter of incentives.

Single-Investigator Versus Consortia-Driven Research

One audience member asked about Omberg's earlier comments about insufficient data when it comes to finding "druggable" targets in addition to the challenges surrounding the use of single-investigator-initiated, hypothesis-driven research, which is often aimed at understanding the fundamental processes of disease rather than just hunting for targets. The audience member questioned whether the best use of a systems approach is to find "druggable" targets or, alternatively, whether it can involve higher priorities such as finding variables that control disease pathway and other preferences. Government-funded research often lacks access to data that come from hospital systems, Omberg replied; in many cases a single institution simply does not have enough data. Consortia can be instrumental for generating larger datasets where multiple academic institutions or industry partners can collaborate to build them. In some cases such collaborative datasets already exist. For example, in mental health research investigating schizophrenia and depression, brain samples often must be collected from brain banks. However, there have been instances where no brain bank had datasets that were sufficient in size to power RNA-sequence analysis or genome-wide association studies analysis. Only by pooling together resources is there enough data, Omberg said.

Single-investigator and consortia-driven research serve different purposes, so neither can replace the other, Omberg said. Systems-level approaches alone are not sufficient to answer all pertinent research questions, so deep dives into individual mechanisms and other inquiries will always be of value, he added. He suggested that individual-investigator- and consortia-driven research approaches be paired, so that systems approaches are supplemented with deep-dive research to better understand and contextualize system-level discoveries. Experiments can then be conducted to validate these approaches.

---

[20] More information about TriNetX is available at https://trinetx.com (accessed December 11, 2020).

As to whether to identify druggable targets or to use more comprehensive approaches to understand disease states—as well as the variables that determine and drive these states—Omberg said that in his collaborative work with AMP AD, they have identified multiple targets. Once a target is identified, certain researchers within AMP AD have advocated for investigating the target's biological basis to better understand its mechanisms and significance. Additionally, the biological investigation of these targets may lead to the discovery of other targets that may be better suited in terms of druggability. Conversely, many pharmaceutical stakeholders have not expressed interest in such biological investigations, Omberg said. Rather, they tend to ask for a target to be identified with the intention of determining its druggability independently. This is an example of divergent views on the importance of these two approaches, he said.

Applying the Concept of Attractor States to Patient Identification

The concept of attractor states (see Chapter 2) may be useful if applied to understand disease processes and inform the identification and stratification of patients at the systems level, Kassim said. Butte proposed using "trajectories of care" to model how patients move through various states within health systems. Related concepts, not yet well explored, include patients' transitions between states, the number of possible states in medicine, and similarities and differences among decision nodes. This modeling work, which is still in its infancy, is complicated because there are no simple trajectories of care to model as a first step. For example, a patient may accumulate multiple conditions or diseases that could each be treated in several different ways. Modeling these types of probabilistic transitions is not a trivial task, Butte said. For instance, acute and chronic diseases would likely be modeled quite differently.

Daily measurements of patients with PD have begun to reveal that patients' response to their medications over time changes over time, Omberg said. In addition, digital biomarker studies have revealed variations between different groups such as between males and females, suggesting a cluster of differences between how biomarkers appeared by gender. Differences were also found between age groups; for example, the response rates to Levodopa varied, with some patients responding in the way they performed a finger tapping test (a measure of bradykinesia), while other had less gait freezing while walking.

Ensuring Patients About Data Security

One audience member commented that patients may seek assurance that their data are secure within health systems such as UCH. Every patient should feel secure, Butte emphasized. The UCH system's primary goal in centralizing its database was "to get patients their own data back," he said. First and foremost, it is for the patients' benefit that their data are organized, harmonized, and entered into tools such as FHIR feeds. Still, it would be tragic if the multi-billion-dollar investments in EHR systems were not also used to improve the practice of medicine, but these improvements must be realized in a safe and respectful manner, Butte said. Because HIPAA has been in place for more than 20 years, managing data under it has become predictable. Those working with patient data know how to de-identify data in accordance with HIPAA; they also have developed research methods for re-introducing certain data elements, such as zip codes, to create "limited datasets," Butte said. The stability of current regulations and policies related to patient data can offer patients assurance that their data are being used in a safe, respectful way. Furthermore, patients sit on UCH institutional review boards and participate in the institutional review process. Researchers and health systems are also subject to the policies of data governance before any patient data—even de-identified patient data—may be exported for any purpose. In cases where there is clearly mutual benefit in sharing de-identified patient data, the contracts used will require that the recipient of the data not re-identify any patients, further protecting patients' data once they have been exported.[21]

In his work related to the DREAM Challenge, Omberg said, he used particular contract language in dealings with the Kaiser Permanente health system, but the contracts were not created with the individuals representing various organizations that participated in the challenge because they did not have access to the data. Challenge participants only agreed to particular requirements, such as making algorithms available using open-source licensing, but their participation did not involve access to patient-identifying data. Setting up contracts such as material transfer agreements or data use agreements can sometimes cause year-long delays because they take time to develop and approve, he added. In some extreme cases data transfers can involve agreements among multiple international and local stakeholders and can take even more than 1 year to finalize. It is always best to harmonize and clean data to minimize complications in data transfers, Omberg said.

Navigating Data Shortcomings

One reason for discussing systems biology, Kassim said, is to enable the systematic identification of quality attributes of products that will lead to clinical responses in regenerative medicine. He asked how data can be

---

[21]Butte remarked on the value of carefully chosen contract language, invoking the term "contract hygiene" to describe the careful crafting of contracts.

used to understand the mechanisms of action or critical quality attributes and whether there are sufficient patient biology, immunology, or product characterization data being collected in the realm of regenerative medicine. Given the mixed nature of datasets—with some data coming from highly regulated analytical methods and other data coming from more exploratory methods—he asked how these data can be integrated into a single database. The amount of data collected will never be sufficient, Omberg said. Researchers must use what data are available and account for the features of those data in their modeling and analysis. Even in cases where sufficient data have ostensibly been captured, rapid changes within biological systems preclude the possibility of maintaining a complete dataset. For example, when a patient has blood drawn at a clinic for omics analysis, that analysis "misses" the patient's entire life history. Thus, the resulting analysis is merely a snapshot. In this sense, researchers will never have enough data. They can, however, use available data to conduct their modeling and analysis, as long as they diligently account for the shortcomings of their datasets. In the face of insufficient data, the task for researchers is to explore what can be done with the data that are currently available, Butte said. Researchers can expect the quality and quantity of data to improve over time, but they should not wait for these improvements. Rather, Butte continued, they should find the best ways to put available data to use.

Behind these data are patients who need to benefit from this research, Butte pointed out—for instance, by using data from the research to identify a patient cohort for enrollment in post-approval studies to acquire molecular markers. Furthermore, residual data from clinical care can be used to study drugs and identify early signs of classifiers for predicting efficacy. Currently, research in regenerative medicine is aimed at predicting success, Butte said. However, introducing real-world evidence can affect early-stage discovery if researchers begin to study failures. For instance, if 30–40 percent of patients are not benefiting from a trial, researchers can enter these patients into a study to measure blood and serum and identify the markers that may be linked to drug failure. He compared this approach to the ways in which smartphone developers rely on bug reports to analyze how and why their technology fails, and suggested that a similar approach to seek out mechanisms of failure is needed in the pharmaceutical and biotechnology industries. Furthermore, those industries would benefit from a new mindset about how data should be used and how research should feed back into the design of products and services, Butte said. He also mentioned the "information commons," which is being deployed across UC campuses as an internal, central repository for data. It includes a cloud-based, secure database where de-identified clinical, imaging, and genomics data can be viewed within the health system by researchers who are in compliance with the requisite data governance processes.

5

Challenges and Opportunities Associated with Systems-Level Analysis and Modeling

Important Points Highlighted by Individual Speakers

- New single-cell RNA sequencing technologies have yielded powerful developments in the capabilities to characterize cell types, link newly uncovered axes of cellular identity to observed phenotypes, and model cell-state transitions using new algorithms. (Fertig)
- Advances in the use of fully spatially resolved single-cell data (i.e., spatial transcriptomics) can now be used to infer cellular interactions within and across the tumor and immune systems. (Fertig)
- Challenges related to interpreting big data, machine learning, and mathematical models and translating into predictions and mechanisms can be addressed by modeling dynamic data to identify a latent space. This approach involves reducing the data's dimensionality in a supervised way that accounts for biological knowledge, modeling the dynamics in low-dimension space, and then re-expanding the models into higher-dimensional space to reconstruct biological properties. (Francois)
- High-throughput methods using high-quality data can precisely quantify and analyze cytokine response through a generative model of cytokine dynamics. Effective two-dimensional dynamics controlled by immune velocity have been found to parsimoniously explain cytokine behavior. However, immune velocity is mostly controlled by antigen strength, and response modulation is related to the characteristics and number of antigen-producing cells. Work is under way to quantitatively assess immune response in immunotherapy. (Francois)

- The application of systems biology and machine learning can help elucidate the relations and dependencies among the multitude of influencing factors along the biopharmaceutical drug development pipeline. This can contribute to producing drugs with the best quality attributes to target diseases as precisely as possible as well as to optimizing the volume and efficiency of drug production while still maintaining efficacy and safety. (Richelle)
- Knowledge gaps and technical limitations that currently restrict the ability to routinely integrate systems biology approaches into the biopharmaceutical product pipeline include (1) an inadequate ability to conduct bioprocess monitoring in real time, (2) the complexity of metabolic networks, and (3) challenges involved in modeling with hybrid approaches. (Richelle)

The fourth session of the workshop focused on challenges and opportunities associated with systems-level analysis and modeling. Malcolm Moos of the Food and Drug Administration (FDA) moderated the session, which featured presentations on the development of algorithms for single cell genomics, modeling dynamic data to identify a latent space, and adapting metabolic modeling tools in biopharmaceutical drug development. This session's objectives were to discuss the current state of the art of systems thinking approaches and talk about how these approaches are being used to inform the identification of important variables to measure and to illuminate current gaps in knowledge and areas for further study.

DEVELOPING ALGORITHMS FOR SINGLE-CELL GENOMICS

Elana Fertig, an associate professor of oncology, biomedical engineering, and applied mathematics and statistics and the associate director of the Convergence Institute at Johns Hopkins University, explored the development of algorithms for single-cell genomics by discussing single-cell technologies, matrix factorization, and other computational techniques. She acknowledged the importance of technological innovation but emphasized the importance of developing computational methods for understanding single-cell genomics as well. She also described some of the needs and challenges involved in developing those computational methods.

Overview of New Single-Cell RNA Technologies

Fertig began with an overview of single-cell technologies by drawing an analogy to different preparations of fruit, comparing the different technologies to smoothies, individual pieces of fruit, and a fruit tart. She compared the previous generation of transcriptional profiling technologies (i.e., bulk RNA sequencing, or RNA-seq) to a fruit smoothie, in that each component of the system is included, but the cellular and molecular components are all blended together to investigate the resulting mixture. In contrast, single-cell RNA-seq can be compared to pieces of fruit, in that each piece of fruit is evaluated individually to observe its molecular state. She likened future single-cell technologies—specifically, spatial transcriptomics—to an elaborate fruit tart. These newer technologies have the potential to reveal not only the presence of each cell, but also the spatial alignment of those cells in a tissue, allowing a system to be characterized in its native context in order to understand its underlying processes. These single-cell RNA technologies are being used to better understand particular cell types involved in these systems, Fertig said. This was previously done using older technologies, such as flow cytometry, but single-cell RNA technologies provide higher-dimensional resolution than their predecessors. She discussed some of these new developments in single-cell RNA technologies related to cell types, axes of cellular identity, and cellular state transitions (Wagner et al., 2016).

Characterizing Cell Types and Axes of Cellular Identity

The single-cell development of the retina across developmental timepoints and cell types has been characterized (Clark et al., 2019; Stein-O'Brien et al., 2019), and Fertig showed a dataset where dots are plotted three-dimensionally to represent individual cells in a retina. The dataset included more than 100,000 cells coded to indicate age and cell type, thus illustrating how the dataset transitions over time. This presentation allows the dataset to be viewed in two ways: either in terms of age or in terms of cell type. Annotation based on these labels limits characterization to a priori knowledge of the system, Fertig said, but the dataset has the power to characterize the entire transcriptional profile of the system beyond just cell types. For example, within each cell type, the single-cell approach can provide information about its phenotype, temporal progression, developmental trajectory, progress along the cell cycle, and spatial position (Wagner et al., 2016).

Encoding this additional information raises the question of how to explore these data in deeper way in order to determine what those phenotypes are, rather than merely clustering or annotating the cells, Fertig said. This question has been addressed in the field of mathematics using matrix factorization (Stein-O'Brien et al., 2018). Using Coordinated Gene Activity in Pattern Sets (CoGAPS), a Bayesian matrix factorization method, a large dataset containing thousands of genes can be analyzed in terms of amplitudes (i.e., gene weights for each biological process) and patterns (i.e., biological processes in each sample) (Fertig et al., 2010). The matrix factorization algorithm finds patterns that define the biological activity in a set of samples (e.g., time points) and the amplitude at which each gene contributes to that biological process. Matrix factorization can be used to learn about the dimensions within a dataset. By linking the results of matrix factorization back to genes or cellular site, it is possible to link back to observed phenotypes, which are fundamental to the system.

Matrix factorization can be applied to uncover the features of cellular identity using the single-cell reference dataset of retinal development, Fertig said (Clark et al., 2019; Stein-O'Brien et al., 2019). She presented a three-dimensional plot showing how some features that undergo the CoGAPS matrix factorization approach reflect individual retina cell types, such as the neurogenic cell type. In addition to learning about cell types—which was already possible with clustering methods—this approach can be used to learn about the fates that reflect changes in cell states. In these three-dimensional Uniform Manifold Approximation and Projection (UMAP) plots with weights of the patterns learned across cells through the matrix factorization, a transition region indicates a space where some cells occur in a pattern that is enriched for cell cycle genes. This pattern is consistent with the desynchronization of the cell cycle, as cells transition from stem cells to developing their final states. By looking across the different axes of this dataset, it is possible to tease out all the different cell types as well as the different transitory states related to age within one algorithm.

Modeling Cell-State Transitions

The inference of cellular state transitions offers a global perspective for observing the system, but the other axes provide more insights into occurrences within the system, Fertig said. Thus, understanding the inference of cell-state transitions and interactions requires new algorithms. Understanding one cell type does not account for additional molecular heterogeneity within that cell type, especially when attempting to understand that variation. Some variation may be associated with cell-state trajectories, such as in stem cells. In addition, there is the challenge of understanding the functioning of these interaction networks and the interaction between cells and molecules that drive phenotypes.

Matrix factorization is not the only approach for modeling cell-state transitions, Fertig said. Indeed, to look at dynamic cell-state transitions, other types of computational methods are more apt. In recent years, two dominant methods have emerged. The first of these is built on the notion of RNA velocity (Melsted et al., 2019), which is based on the idea that the relative maturity of a cell can be calculated by observing the ratio of spliced and unspliced gene products. This information can then be used to determine the cell's trajectory over time, which can be used to calculate the RNA velocity. The other approach relates to trajectory inference, or pseudotime, which involves observing cellular maturity in certain clusters—as well as cells' distances away from each cluster—to determine how the cells change over time and how they are ordered (Trapnell et al., 2014). Each of these metrics can be used to determine a cell's state transitions. These approaches, which use single-cell data, will help move the field through a systems approach that is data-driven but also integrate information about time from dynamic models, Fertig said.

Molecular Heterogeneity with Distinct Cellular Subtypes

Even within a single cell type, temporal changes can be observed, suggesting that there may be additional molecular heterogeneity that can occur within distinct cellular subtypes, Fertig said. Not all cells will use the same pathways at the same level. Moreover, it is not the case that a pathway merely turns on or off in a binary fashion; pathways could be more variable in one state than another. The Expression Variation Analysis method can be used to quantify the degree of difference in variation among transcriptional signatures between cells within one state relative to cells from another (Davis-Marcisak et al., 2019). For example, the variation in expression of cell cycle genes has been found to increase over developmental time in the landmark single-cell retinal development single-cell data, arising from the greater diversity of cell cycle states within the same mature system, Fertig said, rather than the cell cycle simply turning off when mature cell states are obtained (Clark et al., 2019).

Applying Regulatory Algorithms to Uncover Drivers of Cell-State Transitions

Interaction networks can be informed by the genes involved in cell-state transitions or by prior knowledge of biological regulatory networks, Fertig said. These networks can be used to investigate the drivers of cell-state transitions and how a system can become dysregulated by helping to reveal the molecular networks underlying these processes. Two dominant approaches are emerging in this field of inquiry. One approach is based on the idea that knowledge about the trajectories (i.e., how the system is changing over time) can be used to understand the system's causal network in terms of which genes are coming up at specific points over time (Deshpande et al., 2019). The second approach focuses on linking prior molecular knowledge (e.g., gene regulation for ligands and receptors triggering a cascade to transcription factors) with data to understand how those molecular networks are being turned on between cell types (Cherry et al., 2020). These are promising developments because older bulk RNA-seq approaches for understanding these regulatory networks were confounded by intercellular interactions. These new approaches offer a way to discriminate between intercellular and intracellular interactions, Fertig added.

Inferring Cellular Interactions Using Spatial Transcriptomics

Within this broader network-focused perspective, Fertig described a transition in the field from using single-cell data to using fully spatially resolved single-cell data. She showed breast tumor data from a dataset created in collaboration with 10X Genomics using its Visium platform. By annotating the data into separate regions, each region can be spatially resolved into a full transcriptional profile, and matrix factorization can be used to determine the axes of cellular identity in this dataset. This approach makes it possible to differentiate regions in a de novo way in order to identify the dominant signaling processes that distinguish various tumor regions. The same process can be applied within the immune system. Tumor patterns can be linked back to distinct molecular pathways to begin revealing the spatial interactions among tumor and immune systems. In conjunction with network inference algorithms, this approach can provide information about space, time, and regulatory networks. This contributes to the understanding of systems' potential for interaction and of the physical interactions within systems. In closing, Fertig said that single-cell algorithm development is a broad field with much promise. However, new approaches for matrix factorization and latent space analysis are still needed to answer the open questions in the field, such as studying cellular heterogeneity, conducting trajectory and velocity analyses, and identifying network analyses.

MODELING DYNAMIC DATA TO IDENTIFY A LATENT SPACE

Paul Francois, an associate professor in the Department of Physics at McGill University, discussed how dynamic data can be modeled to identify a reduced (i.e., latent) variable space.

Fundamental Challenges

Francois framed the challenges involved in this type of modeling by describing an ideal scenario. Ideally, a high-throughput experimental method could be used to generate data such as mapped representations or complex interaction networks. Then machine learning and mathematical models could be used to generate predictions and reveal the mechanisms or principles of the system's organization. In reality, however, the challenge lies in the translation of big data, machine learning, and mathematics into predictions and mechanisms. Francois described what he calls the "connectionist nightmare," which emerges, for example, when studying protein interaction networks for T cells (Altan-Bonnet and Germain, 2005; Lipniacki et al., 2008). In this case the mathematical modeling of the systems being studied generates numerous equations, making it difficult to understand what is occurring within the system. A similar effect occurs when using deep neural networks to study systems because it is difficult to understand how deep learning and machine learning networks work (Nielsen, 2015). Finally, this effect is related to adversarial examples, in which machine learning is fragile or highly vulnerable to the introduction of noise (Goodfellow et al., 2013). In such examples the introduction of a slight amount of perturbation to a machine learning process may substantially affect the accuracy of the classification algorithm, Francois said.

Another fundamental challenge lies in the interpretation of data and of the impact of how data are plotted or how they are interpreted, Francois said. To demonstrate this point, he invoked the heliocentric and geocentric models of the solar system. Although the heliocentric model is simpler to describe, the geocentric model of the solar system can be plotted using the same data. Similarly, when using an unsupervised method such as UMAP, the UMAP two-dimensional and three-dimensional representations of datasets are different, which raises the question about which representation to choose.[1] The same considerations apply to representations of datasets over time. When researchers are working with complex dynamical systems, they must choose how best to represent movement over time in two dimensions. Francois emphasized the importance of choosing the best way to represent data and the impact of these choices on how researchers think about the problems they study.

General Modeling Approach

Francois described the general approach used to model dynamic data by identifying a latent space. The first step is to take the data and reduce its dimensionality in a supervised way—which accounts for biological knowledge—using tailored algorithms, such as a reduction algorithm that reduces large networks (Proulx-Giraldeau et al., 2017). Evolutionary algorithms and auto-encoders can also be applied to understand biological data and identify the most relevant features within datasets (Beaupeux and François, 2016; Henry et al., 2018). Once the dimensionality of the complex dynamical system has been reduced, its dynamics can be modeled in low-dimension space. Low-dimension models are easier to study, and one can derive more general results there (e.g., theorems can be more easily proven). Models can

---

[1] More information about UMAP is available at https://umap-learn.readthedocs.io/en/latest (accessed November 23, 2020).

Generative Model of Cytokine Dynamics

This general approach has been applied to develop a generative model of cytokine dynamics, Francois said (Altan-Bonnet and Mukherjee, 2019). T cells interact in the immune system and produce cytokines which determine how the cell reacts to antigens. From that point there are numerous possibilities with various outcomes, Francois said. Next, the antigen concentration or the number of T cells can be varied, to generate IL-2 (a cytokine), which can rise or fall depending on the situation. Many other dimensions or parameters involved in this system can be manipulated to investigate cytokine dynamics. Francois highlighted the importance of ligand strength as a biochemical parameter within cytokine dynamics. Ligand strength affects immunotherapy because the immune response depends on ligand strength.

Francois and his colleagues developed a stepwise process with multiple readouts that uses a robot to study immune response in vitro at multiple time-points. The process begins with harvesting primary immune cells, after which mixtures of T cells and antigen-presenting cells (APCs) mixtures are prepared. Next the robot collects time series data, which are processed along with data collected via flow cytometer. The pipeline currently follows 7 cytokines and 12 markers and takes data at 12 time points, with 50,000 cells per condition. The result is a reliable and precisely generated map of the ways in which T cells react in the test tube in the presence of different antigens. This process generates highly multidimensional data, which are modeled using new techniques developed by Francois and colleagues, including evolutionary algorithms.

Reducing Dimensionality in a Supervised Way

Francois also described the process of reducing dimensionality in a supervised way that accounts for biological knowledge. The first step, he said, is finding the right variables. An evolutionary algorithm was used to find the variables and suggested an integral of the natural logs of cytokines. Indeed, analyzing three-dimensional plots of data from three cytokines reveals that plots of integral logs visually appear as the best way to disentangle and represent the data. This choice about how to best represent data is analogous to the choice about whether to represent planetary motion data using a heliocentric or geocentric model, he said. Using the representation of the data involving plots of integral logs shows a consistent trajectory of the various antigens being studied in the integral-of-log space. Next, classical machine learning methods can be used to project the trajectories of the resulting plot and classify antigens based on ligand strength.

Modeling Dynamics in Low-Dimension (Latent) Space

This process of reducing dimensionality in a supervised way can be used to model cytokine dynamics in low-dimension space, Francois said. The trajectory can be modeled in two dimensions by using physics to model the dynamics. In the reduced (or "latent") space, ballistic physics equations appear as a convenient way to parameterize the cytokine curves in order to describe the trajectories using these parameters. It was found that all the parameters correlated with each other, which means the complicated trajectories of cytokines can be modeled with a single parameter, which is essentially the initial slope. This parameter is called *immune velocity* because it is connected to the initial angle of the trajectory and the way it will decrease.

Re-Expanding the Model to Explain Biology

Once the high-dimensional system has been reduced and modeled in low-dimensional space, it is possible to begin testing hypotheses, Francois said. For instance, the data that were not used to train the model can be fed into the parameters of the model to test whether the model works. In the case of immune velocity, probing the correlation between time and initial immune velocity reveals an appropriate structure in the data. New antigens are entered into the system and layered intermittently between other antigens in order to predict the trends of those new antigens. Furthermore, the complete mathematical model of the cytokine response generated upon expanding back to the biological data can be applied back to understand a specific aspect of the original data, such as IL-2, in order to connect immune velocity to parameters of the curve (e.g., cutoff time). This type of process led to the discovery of the innate versus adaptive cytokine parameter, he added. An entire ensemble of connections between cytokines was discovered using this dimensional reduction process by employing the simple parameter of immune velocity.

Major Findings and Ways Forward in Applying the Model

In conclusion, Francois reiterated that high-throughput methods using high-quality data can be used to precisely quantify and analyze cytokine response. The challenge is determining the best means to render the data in two dimensions using evolutionary algorithms in a supervised manner to refine the data and determine the immune velocity. Effective two-dimensional dynamics controlled by immune velocity have been found to parsimoniously explain all cytokine behavior, but immune velocity is mostly controlled by antigen strength, and the modulation of the response is related to the nature of APCs and the number of cells. Francois noted that there is work under way to apply this approach to assessing immune response quantitatively in immunotherapy.

ADOPTING METABOLIC MODELING TOOLS IN BIOPHARMACEUTICAL DRUG DEVELOPMENT

Anne Richelle, a senior specialist on metabolic modeling at GlaxoSmithKline, explored the adoption of metabolic modeling tools in the biopharmaceutical industry. She discussed how systems thinking can be applied to strengthen the global drug production pipeline and discussed challenges related to implementing systems thinking in the biopharmaceutical industry.

Timeline of Drug Development

Richelle began by describing the typical timeline of research activities in drug development. The process begins with studying a disease, with a focus on drug discovery and target identification. Emergent technologies are used to identify a host organism to be engineered. The aim of this step is to identify or engineer a host cell that will be able to produce the best drug that has quality attributes that enable the disease to be targeted as precisely as possible. During the process development phase, host organisms are cultivated in controlled conditions to create an optimal environment for producing the drug. Finally, this process is scaled up during the manufacturing phase in order to produce as much of the drug as possible—as quickly as possible—while still maintaining efficacy and safety.

This is a simplified timeline of the drug development pipeline, Richelle noted; in reality, there are many additional barriers and subprocesses that greatly influence analyses and development processes at every step of the way. For instance, a patient's genetics, sex, and age can influence the expression of disease and the molecular interactions identified in the prospective drug. Moreover, host organisms have their own genetic attributes that can influence protein or molecule attributes. However, the proper interaction between the target and the drug is defined based on these conformational attributes and can strongly influence the efficacy of the drug. Environmental factors can also affect the development process. If the environment is not optimal, it can influence the genetic expression of the host organism, which in turn influences the protein and molecule quality attributes that determine the drug's therapeutic ability to treat the target disease.

Large amounts of data are collected during the development process to monitor and manipulate these types of influencing factors, Richelle said. In her opinion, she said, the biopharma sector as it currently stands is far from being "big data." Instead, she described the data generated in the biopharma field as "low and expensive" and often not easily accessible in machine-readable format[2] (Richelle and von Stosch, 2020). Furthermore, the lack of standardization in the existing databases (e.g., varying nomenclatures, the heterogeneity of the experimental methods and analysis methods resulting in many hidden variables) makes them difficult to exploit without extensive processing. With the digital transformation occurring in this sector, biopharmaceutical researchers are now faced with finding ways to integrate these diverse data sources and extract meaningful information. These challenges might take a decade to resolve, she added, but hopefully it will be less with the emergence of new technologies in this field.

Machine Learning as a Driver of Discovery

Machine learning is a powerful tool that helps researchers in all fields extract information from data, Richelle said. Some sectors are positioned for greater gains from the use of big data, while other fields may not see the same benefits. The benefits of machine learning depend on the relationship between the amount of data available and the impact of exploiting those data (Manyika et al., 2011). For instance, Richelle said, machine learning has been applied successfully in the fields of personalized marketing, in which the potential impact of exploiting the large volume of available data is relatively high. In the case of using machine learning to optimize bioprocess development, the potential impact of exploiting data is relatively high, but the amount of data available is relatively low. Still, even though the volume of available data is relatively low, machine learning will likely have a substantial impact on the biopharmaceutical pipeline, Richelle predicted. But large datasets "cannot speak for themselves," especially when those datasets contain randomness that may result in spurious correlations due to non-causal coincidences, hidden factors, or the nature of big randomness (Calude and Longo, 2017). Furthermore, many of the algorithms used in machine learning are difficult to carefully scrutinize during peer review, for example. According to research by Patrick Riley, "many of the algorithms [used in machine learning] are so complicated that it is impossible to inspect all parameters or to reason about how exactly the inputs have been manipulated" (Riley, 2019, p. 27). Richelle added that typical machine learning processes are like black boxes: although they may be instrumental

---

[2] Richelle noted that the work being done to mine the world's research papers (Pulla, 2019) might change the way to extract information from historical studies.

in developing predictive models, they do not provide explanations for their results. To address this challenge, she suggested that the body of empirical knowledge that has been developed in the field of biology should be incorporated into efforts to apply machine learning to drug development.

Applying Systems Biology to Drug Development

The factors that influence the drug development process are related and interdependent, Richelle said. These relations and dependencies need to be considered—including the feedback effects among these factors—in applying the systems thinking approach to observe the network of interconnected influence factors and to alter that network. Altering such networks is generally done to achieve three outcomes: (1) producing as much of the drug as possible, (2) producing the drug as quickly as possible, and (3) producing a drug that all data suggest is the best product to cure the targeted disease. Systems biology typically uses a network-based approach to organize large datasets and glean insights about complex biological systems, Richelle said. Coherently organizing large datasets into biological networks can provide non-intuitive insights on biological systems that in vivo experiments alone cannot provide. Network-based approaches also offer a platform for integrating and interpreting omics data to explore links between genotype and phenotype. For instance, this approach has been used to map metabolic networks and integrate data sources.

The systems biology approach can reveal more than just a network of reactions; it can generate an interconnected map of cellular functions. This approach has been used to develop algorithms that recapitulate the metabolism of specific cell and tissue types, offering useful insights into metabolic activity under these conditions, Richelle said (Opdam et al., 2017). These systems tools have proven to be invaluable at the level of preclinical research, she said. For example, in designing new drugs, the tools can be used to inform target selection and to make it possible to engineer cells to rewire their metabolism toward the production of a product of interest. While the systems thinking approach has brought much value to the study and manipulation of biological networks, it also has potential to be applied to many other influence factors across the drug development pipeline, Richelle said. The tools of systems thinking can be used for process design, monitoring, and control. They can also be applied to lower experimental effort, increase process robustness, and facilitate the implementation of regulatory requirements, such as quality-by-design and process analytical tools (Richelle et al., 2020).

Knowledge Gaps and Technical Limitations

Metabolic modeling tools can be used in drug development to expedite the process and integrate existing knowledge regarding the target disease, the protein, or the molecule being produced and the host organism, Richelle said. However, she highlighted three areas in which gaps in knowledge and technical limitations currently restrict the routine integration of systems biology tools into the biopharmaceutical product pipeline: (1) real-time bioprocess monitoring, (2) the complexity of metabolic networks, and (3) modeling with hybrid approaches (Richelle et al., 2020).

Real-Time Bioprocess Monitoring

Real-time monitoring technologies are a critical aspect of automation, Richelle said. Current data collection methods are unable to acquire real-time in situ measurements of metabolites and cell concentrations, which limits the ability to take a "live snapshot" of cell metabolism. Although there is increasing interest in spectroscopic methods (e.g., near-infrared spectroscopy, Fourier-transform infrared, mid-infrared, Raman, fluorescence) that can capture a "molecular fingerprint" of samples, the current capacity to systematically extract accurate quantitative data is limited to a handful of metabolites. She noted, however, that advances in the chemometric modeling field will contribute to developing methods to effectively extract maximum information from these types of spectra. Furthermore, advances in online single-cell probing are ushering in a new generation of high-throughput omics technologies. Richelle speculated that near-real-time measurements of cell transcriptomes and proteomes may be available relatively soon.

Complexity of Metabolic Networks

The complexity of metabolic networks limits the ability to make predictions, Richelle said. Furthermore, the complexity of large networks hinders their utility in practical applications. For example, solving large metabolic networks will require large quantities of data. Otherwise the systems will be underdetermined, leading to a multitude of alternative yet equivalent solutions to a given problem. Therefore, these types of complex networks are not often used to develop feedback control and optimize processes. Various approaches have been proposed for tailoring metabolic networks based on a priori knowledge or available experimental data. However, it is difficult to define the data to be used and determine how to overlay these data on the network. This problem is highlighted by the open question in biology about the links between genes, proteins, and metabolites and how to define the phenotype that should be "protected" during the reduction. Due to the lack of a quantitative description of the gene–protein–reaction rule, strong assumptions are needed to link gene expression and metabolic reaction activity. Moreover, network-tailoring approaches typically do not completely solve the problem of system underdetermination; thus, the choice of an adequate strategy to solve the system will always be required to achieve an instantaneous picture of the flux distributions in the cell. Ultimately, shortages of mathematicians that work on these complex problems is also a limiting factor, Richelle said.

Modeling with Hybrid Approaches

Further challenges relate to modeling with hybrid approaches, Richelle said. Interest is increasing in the use of machine learning and artificial intelligence for bioprocessing and engineering, such as technologies that use digital imaging for automated counting of cell colonies grown on petri dishes (Ferrari et al., 2017). Using machine learning and artificial intelligence tools for bioprocessing and engineering could be a powerful approach and may potentially inform control and optimization strategies as it could be used to establish relationship between metabolism and operating conditions that cannot yet be mechanistically explained. Many aspects of complexity cannot be explained with mechanistic descriptions, Richelle noted. This approach can contribute to resolving the complexity within the "black box" of machine learning and artificial intelligence, she suggested. However, this approach would require more applications that combine artificial intelligence and machine learning with the tools of biology, a dedicated software approach, and interdisciplinary experts with broad skill sets working on the problem. Several major open questions related to pursuing these approaches also remain unaddressed, such as how to effectively generate sufficiently informative experimental data and how to identify joint parameters across the mechanistic and data-driven parts of the model. In closing, Richelle emphasized that advancing the field toward so-called "biopharma 4.0" would benefit from a more global approach that applies machine learning to reveal interactions among factors that influence the drug production pipeline.

DISCUSSION

Dimensionality of Biological Systems

The panel discussion began with a comment from Moos on the theme of reducing dimensionality, and he referred the audience to Huang's earlier discussion about the characterization of cell state in terms of a state vector.

Early on, it was suggested that the vector would need to contain 2,000 to 3,000 elements in order to fully describe a cell transcriptome (Huang et al., 2005). Moos asked whether that number of elements is necessary to convey most of the information, because (1) many of those elements are not relevant to the distinction between states and (2) some of the elements could be collapsed into simpler signal transduction pathway elements. Work on factorization approaches has begun to reveal that the dimensionality is a function of the biology that researchers are trying to capture, Fertig said, so there are no right or wrong dimensions. Instead, the focus is on the dimension that the research is trying to uncover in the system. In the days of bulk RNA-sequencing, researchers found that by representing two dimensions in a system it was possible to separate tumor from normal tissue. By increasing the number of dimensions it was possible to separate various tumor subtypes (Fertig et al., 2013). Fertig added that the hierarchy of dimensions in biological systems likely warrants a hierarchy of methods—in terms of multi-scale dimensionality—to uncover a system (Way et al., 2020). This suggests that the systems are fundamentally low dimensional but multi-scale, depending on which dimension the work is trying to capture. Furthermore, various computational methodologies will yield different dimensions or features, requiring different latent space methods based on the target dimension researchers are trying to uncover.

Accounting for Zeros in Datasets

A technical issue related to sampling can arise when a zero appears in a data matrix, and speakers were asked if that means "no expression" or "dropout." Relatively few efforts have explicitly addressed this question, Moos said, although Fabian Theis and colleagues have started to do so using an autoencoder. The pipeline developed by Francois and his colleagues allows for multiple repeated experiments to account for these types of problems with data points, he said. This and other aspects of their process allow researchers to maintain some amount of quality control when data points are missing. Francois's team can use their dataset to correct for missing data points in a reasonable and coherent way, either by accounting for the missing data points or by using them to show that the experiment has not worked. Unlike single-cell RNA sequencing, this method can systematically evaluate many dimensions of the same data point.

For sampling reasons, researchers may not capture all of the potentially useful elements when using semi-supervised methods to search for the presence or absence of an activated signal transduction pathway, Moos said. He asked whether the one-or-zero issue might be a logistic regression problem that, in a neural-network approach, could help determine whether a neuron has fired. Embedding architecture into systems might help elucidate where things are occurring or not, Fertig said. Even factorization approaches can reveal different features depending on the prior knowledge encoded into the factorized genes. This multi-scale nature of systems is critical for understanding the processes involved, she said. A long-standing issue in genomics research is that the depth of knowledge generated depends on the depth of research focused on, for example, a specific cell type. In genomics, the data analysis should be just as hypothesis-driven as the experiment if the aim is to uncover some phenomenon, she emphasized.

Insights About Biologic Processes from the Projection Space

The projection space that works for visualizations of data correlations also provides insight into the biologic process or network, Francois said. For example, the manifold where data are projected is related to the relative magnitude of two broad types of cytokines, the ones more associated to innate responses versus the ones more associated to adaptive responses. This requires further explanation, she said, because there is likely to be interesting biological information where this low-dimension manifold sits, which might vary between different antigens and T cell receptors.

Using Immune Velocity to Phenotype Immune Health

The possibility of using immune velocity to phenotype a patient's immune health is an area that is still being explored, Francois said. It has not yet reached the stage where it is possible to look at what happens to patients based on their age, gender, and pre-existing conditions, he said. Currently, he and his colleagues are looking at different T cells and T cell receptors to see how immune velocity is defined. He and his team have found that immune velocity is a property of the antigen itself and that the approach can also be applied to other types of immune cells. He was optimistic that the tool he developed with his colleagues would eventually allow for quantifying those properties in various contexts. Moos asked whether immune velocity may be used as a functional test (e.g., for immune system–directed cellular cancer therapy). This is precisely what his group is aiming to achieve with their work, Francois replied.

Optimization in Process Design

Given that many developmental processes are modular by nature, Moos asked if the concept of sequential attractor states might help to simplify process design. A more global perspective would be helpful, Richelle said, but framing all processes as single, unitary operations is also problematic. She cautioned that focusing exclusively on optimizing every step in a drug development process (e.g., in pursuit of optimal conditions for an organism) can risk one overlooking the direct impact of these optimizations on the drug itself. Optimization efforts should consider the influence of that optimization on the molecule being produced and how that affects the efficacy of the drug. Solutions that initially seem suboptimal may actually be optimal for treating the disease, she added.

Hybrid Models of Machine Learning and Biological Systems

Many researchers are moving toward the combination of machine learning and the study of biological systems, sometimes called the hybrid model, Richelle said. However, there is more than one way to consider and integrate these two approaches. For example, in studying the influence of temperature on metabolism, some researchers might introduce numerous kinetic parameters to see how they affect each metabolic reaction, while others might try to combine these parameters into a single statistical effect. There is no one right approach, as different approaches fit different purposes: for instance, she said, developing a very complex model to describe the influence of the temperature on the metabolism at the metabolic reaction level might be conceptually interesting, but less useful for controlling and developing a process. The precise way that data-driven approaches are merged with systems biology will need to depend on the purpose of the merging.

Patient-Focused Biological Systems Approach

In thinking about a biological systems approach, it may be useful to consider if it can begin with a patient, Moos said. Although a patient represents a sample of one, each individual hosts many complex, interacting biological activities. Given the aim of developing a broadly successful suite of therapies, it might be worthwhile to position iterative regenerative drug development processes so that they begin by distinguishing patients who respond from patients who do not. Modeling should begin at the level of disease, and the disease should be a focus throughout the process, Richelle said. A model that is person-specific could be used to explore parallel patient-specific factors (e.g., genetics, age, gender) that influence the development of personalized medicines, thus providing opportunities to expedite the development process. One goal would be to use a patient's DNA sample to evaluate how the disease is manifesting in that patient. This information could be used to appropriately target the specific quality attributes of a molecule that would allow the disease to be targeted most efficiently in that patient. Theoretically, understanding the interactions among those factors could be used to rapidly produce a molecule that is targeted uniquely for the specific patient's expression of the disease, Richelle said.

Clustering Algorithms Versus Matrix Factorization

Many methods for identifying different cell types are based on clustering algorithms that treat all transcripts identically, Moos said, even though the determination of one cell fate over another may not depend on, for example, whether it is expressing aldolase and whether Bmp or Wnt signaling have been activated. Classical algorithms for comparing protein sequences recognize that changing an aspartate for a glutamate is not nearly as consequential as changing an aspartate for a phenylalanine. However, few clustering methods incorporate that recognition. Moos asked how this limitation of existing clustering methods might be addressed. Fertig said that these concerns have motivated her work with latent space representations and matrix factorization, rather than clustering methods, because the former approaches allow for gene reuse. A major limitation of clustering algorithms is that genes are forced to be a member of one class or another, despite the knowledge that genes are reused for multiple processes, as demonstrated by biological systems and systems-level approaches. This is a major advantage of matrix factorization over clustering, she added. Fertig and colleagues are exploring a transfer-learning approach to benchmark transitions from one cell type to another in datasets in which there is a known "ground truth" of a particular cell type. This avoids the reliance on a single gene; rather, it involves looking at gene signatures and how they are preserved across datasets and across cell types, she added.

Impact of Scale and Function Within a Single Transcript

Fertig also discussed that impact of scale and function within a single transcript, which is often ignored even in matrix factorization techniques. Her CoGAPS approach explicitly encodes the uncertainty in each matrix element as a variable. This allows for scaling how much that transcripts express, which can then be down-weighed to avoid bias toward the most highly expressed transcripts. This semi-supervised learning approach may be powerful if various features can be encoded into the system. Furthermore, she added, it may help researchers understand the relevant factors without introducing bias toward the most highly expressed or most correlated genes. The dominance of elements that are abundant rather than important (e.g., comparing transcripts for structural proteins versus receptors and transcription factors) is a limitation in this work that has not received adequate attention, Moos said. Certain practices, such as zero mean and unit variance, continue to endure despite the knowledge that important genes are being regulated in a bistable manner. He asked how this trend may be connected to the idea that multi-omics data—if they too are regulated in a bistable manner—may be amenable to simple scaling as 1s and 0s. Fertig said that this has been considered in terms of weighing down the system by the uncertainty matrix as well as by modeling regulation in a specific manner. The varying error terms in different modalities can then be included in an integrated framework. It can be useful to follow a smaller number of genes by repeating the same experiment over time, Francois added, because following a trajectory over time can reveal interesting geometric features in the data. If different experiments conducted at different times are compared, noise emerges that might not be controllable. Francois also commented on the critical period of transition between the monostable and bistable phase, during which a set of cells can be followed as a function of time. Following the entire trajectory can also reveal interesting features. The critical period of time between phase transitions is crucial in studying and modeling developmental systems, he emphasized.

6

Addressing Regenerative Medicine Manufacturing and Supply Chain Challenges with Systems-Level Approaches

Important Points Highlighted by Individual Speakers

- Deep-learning artificial intelligence capabilities make it possible to harness and automate the analysis of data from multiple sources and apply those abilities in the field of cell and gene therapy to (1) generate breakthrough discoveries; (2) empower scientists, clinicians, and citizen scientists; (3) learn cause and effect from data; (4) glean insights to optimize manufacturing; (5) predict patient outcomes; and (6) build a "system of intelligence" for the development of cell and gene therapies. (Khalil, Tyagarajan)
- In the discovery and development process for new therapies, a dynamic sampling platform can help to optimize experimental process parameters and develop a multi-omics integrative approach for early predictive signatures. (Kotanchek)
- Collections of models with greater accuracy and lower complexity can be used to build "ensembles" of accurate-fit, trustable models to guide decision making and enable active learning and active design of experiments. (Kotanchek)
- Digital modeling and simulation of supply chain and manufacturing process are efficient and cost-effective approaches to (1) build a decision-support toolset for supply chain design, planning, and control; (2) develop and validate models of manufacturing and quality assurance; (3) inform standards and regulatory development; and (4) support workforce development. (Wang)
- A systems approach to digital modeling and simulation in manufacturing can be applied to support capacity planning, inform strategies to manage supply chain disruptions and demand surges, and model costs of production and automation. (Wang)

The fifth session of the workshop focused on addressing regenerative medicine manufacturing and supply chain challenges with systems-level approaches. The session was moderated by Krishnendu Roy, the Robert A. Milton Chair Professor, the director of the National Science Foundation's (NSF's) Engineering Research Center for Cell Manufacturing Technologies (CMaT), and the director of the Marcus Center for Therapeutic Cell Characterization and Manufacturing at the Wallace H. Coulter Department of Biomedical Engineering at the Georgia Institute of Technology and Emory University. The session featured presentations on using artificial intelligence (AI) in cell and gene therapies, in modeling manufacturing processes in regenerative medicine, and in modeling the supply chain and other processes involved in cell therapy manufacturing and distribution. The session's objective was to highlight opportunities where systems thinking approaches could address inefficiencies with manufacturing and the supply chain related to regenerative medicine.

ARTIFICIAL INTELLIGENCE IN CELL AND GENE THERAPIES

Iya Khalil, the global head of the AI Innovation Center, and Seshu Tyagarajan, the global head of Late Stage CMC Strategy, Cell and Gene Therapies, Novartis Technical Operations, both at Novartis, provided an overview of current work with AI for manufacturing cell and gene therapies, outlining how they are approaching and solving problems and the types of data they are using in this process.

New Opportunities to Apply Artificial Intelligence

The possibilities of AI are being realized in many fields, Khalil said, whether in building a disease model from omics data or understanding a particular medicine's manufacturing or supply chain process or some other application. The reason for the use of AI in so many fields, she added, is the unprecedented ability today to collect all kinds of data, including measures on the patient level, on the granular level of a genomic, molecular, or phenotypic screen readout, or actual health outcomes at a single point of time or over time. It also includes knowledge about how to generate an effective cell therapy or immune drug. The ability to collect all of these data, coupled with advances in AI, creates the potential for new learning (Topol, 2019). Deep learning algorithms are a class of AI algorithms that can be applied to discern complex patterns underlying the data, Khalil said. As more data are fed into those algorithms, the potential for accurate algorithms increases, exceeding what was possible with machine learning 5 to 10 years ago, Khalil said. Combined with the capabilities of computational power, these advances in AI contribute to strengthening the overall ability to learn from data, make predictions from data, and reason based on those data.

Using Deep Learning Algorithms to Detect Diabetic Retinopathy

Khalil provided examples of how this process is being applied to diabetic macular degeneration as it relates to follow-on diseases such as diabetic retinopathy. Starting with retinal images, high-performance supercomputing and AI can be used to achieve promising outcomes and develop new knowledge from the data that previously could not be accessed. For example, results from an algorithm for detecting diabetic retinopathy and macular edema were comparable to the capabilities of ophthalmologists (Gulshan et al., 2016). Beyond matching or potentially exceeding ophthalmologists' diagnostic abilities, algorithms are also finding new associations beyond imaging data. They are, for example, combining imaging data with biomarker data in an effort to learn how macular degeneration might impact outcomes, such as adverse cardiac events (Poplin et al., 2018). In 2018 an AI-based diabetic retinopathy diagnostic system was approved by the Food and Drug Administration (FDA), so this algorithm can now be applied at the point of care (Abràmoff et al., 2018). These developments demonstrate what can potentially be achieved with AI and data, Khalil said.

Harnessing Core Artificial Intelligence Capabilities

Khalil said that her group is working on harnessing core AI capabilities that involve deep learning and that extend to approaches involving causal learning. Data are harnessed from a variety of sources, including text and files analyzed using natural language processing (NLP) and image analytics, such as readouts of flow data from manufacturing processes. AI is applied to an automated analysis—so that it is no longer a tedious job for humans—and combined with advances in visual analytics.

Applying Artificial Intelligence to Drive Exploration and Empowerment

Together, these combined advances in capabilities allow for more than just an in-depth look at one AI field, Khalil said. Her group is applying these capabilities in two different ways: (1) AI exploration for breakthrough discoveries and (2) AI empowerment of citizen scientists. Exploration involves gaining a solid understanding of the fundamental mechanisms and processes that drive what is observed and the outcomes that are being modeled. Empowerment involves creating capabilities not only for the deep-data AI scientists who know how to use these tools, but also for the data scientists—and even non-data scientists—who want to improve their abilities to interact and reason with data. Harnessing the power and potential of AI is important, Khalil said, because it can drive fundamental discoveries and empower scientists and clinicians throughout an organization. She briefly shared examples of applications of AI, including applying visual analytics methods to flow cytometry data (Bachthaler and Weiskopf, 2008; Ray and Pyne, 2012). Beyond analyzing images, Khalil's team is also gaining insights from unstructured data. They achieve these insights by using NLP capabilities to analyze massive amounts of corpus text data and automating the ability to learn and extract adverse FDA events from text data and apply this to drug labels (Ly et al., 2018). Insights can also be extracted from electronic health record (EHR) data, a task that formerly required the deployment of many people to pull data from NLP records and EHRs. However, various AI and NLP methods can scale this quickly, making it much easier and more straightforward to use the data from EHRs to predict treatment outcomes (Liu et al., 2019).

Applying Artificial Intelligence to Learn Cause and Effect from Data

Another fundamental capability harnessed specifically in cell and gene therapy is the ability to learn cause and effect from data, Khalil said. One data approach is to try to learn these complex patterns from the space between inputs and outputs, which Khalil described as a "bit of a black box." Another approach is to strive for transparency and a better understanding of the underlying processes in the system that gave rise to the data. Through causal learning and graphical causal learning methods, it is now possible to analyze datasets that include sets of inputs that modulate responses in the system and then learn how these factors form a causal network that can be mapped out and whose behavior can be predicted (Schadt et al., 2005). This causal network demonstrates influences on outcomes (e.g., whether the nodes being measured are causal for the outcome or reactive to the outcome). Developing the capability to perform a "sorting of causality" is helpful in addressing confounding factors, which are major underlying issues with these types of datasets. For instance, if only large-scale patterns of associations in datasets are evaluated, it can lead to the incorrect inference that insulin and amputation are merely associated, when in fact there is an underlying cause: the confounding factor that having diabetes will influence changes in insulin levels, which can influence the possibility of amputation. Therefore, it is actually diabetes, not insulin, that is directly associated with amputation. Underlying statistical and mathematical probabilities allow cause and effect to be sorted out mathematically, she added. Technology has been developed for learning cause-and-effect associations not only at a small graphical level, but also at scale.

Other AI capabilities are being used in cell and gene therapy across different data modalities and types that allow work with imaging data, NLP data, and sorting out cause and effect. There is a huge potential, Khalil said, to learn to identify the various key steps in the complex manufacturing process for patient-specific cell therapy, starting with the patient, then applying treatment and cell therapy into the patient, and finally monitoring the patient long-term, collecting a variety of data modalities throughout the process. A goal is to learn how AI and machine learning models can be applied to understand the manufacturing process, then determine how to intervene to optimize those processes.

Cell and Gene Therapy: Supporting the End-to-End Patient Journey

The long-term vision and mission of cell and gene therapy development at Novartis is to understand the end-to-end patient journey as fully as possible, Tyagarajan said. The goal is to improve every step along that journey (e.g., understanding and improving the incoming material can aid in better patient selection, which in turn can lead to improvements in robust manufacturing). Consequently, these advances could reduce vein-to-vein time, improve predictability, and ultimately enable the product to reach a greater patient population. She acknowledged that cell and gene therapy is a nascent field with many challenges, such as process variability, donor-to-donor variability, availability of raw materials, a shortage of analytical assays, a need for analytical development, limited choice of vendors, logistics and supply chain issues, a shortage of trained personnel, and rapid timelines. Thus, she said, she and her colleagues are always looking for ways to learn more about the patient journey so that processes can be expedited and barriers removed.

Developing Autologous Cell Therapies

The process of developing autologous chimeric antigen receptor (CAR) T cell therapy begins with cell collection from the patient, Tyagarajan explained. The patient's T cells are selected, modified, expanded, formulated, frozen, and sent back to the patient for treatment via infusion. A systems approach is used to identify the factors that influence each data-collection point in the process: patient characteristics, apheresis, manufacturing, final product, cellular kinetics, and outcome (see Table 6-1). Because each step affects the next step or steps, there are dependencies involved that are not well understood. Multiple datasets are collected at each stage, including various types of patient data, apheresis information, extensive manufacturing information, product measurements, cellular kinetics data,

TABLE 6-1 Factors Influencing Each Stage in the Development of Autologous Cell Therapies

Data-Collection Stage	Considerations
Patient	• Disease stage • Disease burden • Prior treatments • Patient fitness • Molecular subtypes
Apheresis	• Cell composition (e.g., monocytes, blastocytes, T cells) • T cell activation and maturation (e.g., senescence, exhaustion)
Manufacturing	• Raw materials • Day 0 pathway • Growth rate • Population-doubling level • Cell-penetrating peptides • Induced pluripotent stem cells • Harvest • Cryopreservation
Final product	• Dose • Purity • Transduction • Viability • T cell phenotypes • T cell function • T cell potency
Cellular kinetics	• Expansion • Persistence • In vivo phenotype • Distribution
Outcome	• Efficacy • Safety (e.g., cytokine release syndrome) • Durability of response

SOURCE: Seshu Tyagarajan workshop presentation, October 23, 2020.

and pharmacokinetics and pharmacodynamics information. AI is used to derive answers from these datasets, she added.

Advancing the Field of Cell and Gene Therapy

There are three research questions Novartis is pursuing to implement AI in the burgeoning field of cell and gene therapy, Tyagarajan said. These include (1) how to achieve a better understanding of the cell and gene therapy manufacturing process by identifying the factors that are most important, (2) whether those factors and their associated data can be used to predict clinical outcomes, and (3) how to rapidly translate lessons from these initial explorations into the next generation of clinical trials. She outlined some of the strategies Novartis is using to address these questions.

To achieve a better understanding of the factors that are important for manufacturing, Tyagarajan and her colleagues are analyzing available data by combining them into multiple datasets. One set of data is coalesced into the patient group, another set into the apheresis group, and others into the manufacturing dataset and the final product dataset. The goal of coalescing these datasets is to predict the out-of-sample value of a node in the graph in order to identify the individual factors important for manufacturing a better product. To determine whether these factors can be used to predict patient outcomes, the number of influencing factors is increased to identify other factors that may be confounding. Dose and final product characteristics are added to the first group of datasets with the goal of identifying how these factors influence response and how the nodes in the graph interact with each other. The aims of this process are to (1) identify confounders of the problem, (2) create a model to predict response with dose and confounders, and (3) develop a way to marginalize out the confounders. Confounders between dose and response can include patient characteristics (e.g., body mass index, age, tumor size) and product characteristics.

The next step in the process involves grouping data, applying machine learning models, and learning from random forest analysis to build a system of intelligence. The system of intelligence is composed of a user interface, a data ingestion pipeline of clinical and other datasets, and a knowledge ingestion pipeline of medical and biological knowledge. Statistics, machine learning, and cloud computing are applied to all of the system's components to yield insights that must then be validated. Creating this system of intelligence for cell and gene therapy is in its early stages, having commenced only a year ago, but Tyagarajan said that much work is taking place during this promising stage of development.

MODELING THE MANUFACTURING PROCESS IN REGENERATIVE MEDICINE

Theresa Kotanchek, the chief executive officer of Evolved Analytics, LLC, highlighted notable challenges in cell manufacturing, various modeling processes to address those challenges, and recent projects and achievements.

Grand Challenges in Cell Manufacturing

Kotanchek opened by briefly listing eight grand challenges in the field of cell manufacturing (see Box 6-1). NSF's CMaT was formed to address

> **BOX 6-1**
> **Grand Challenges in Cell Manufacturing**
>
> - Addressing the lack of reproducibility, standards, and quality-by-design
> - Identifying the quality attributes that make a cell safe and effective, determining what to measure, and pinpointing which cells are considered "good" in the midst of heterogeneity
> - Determining how to measure critical quality attributes in line and during manufacturing
> - Developing methods to grow billions of safe and potent cells from a patient or donor
> - Predicting the safety and potency for specific indications and patients
> - Purifying, storing, freezing, and transporting cells without compromising their quality
> - Achieving end-to-end manufacturing of a high-quality product at a low cost
> - Addressing the lack of a trained cell manufacturing workforce
>
> SOURCES: Theresa Kotanchek workshop presentation, October 23, 2020. Adapted from NCMC, 2016.

such challenges with the vision of transforming the manufacture of cell-based therapeutics into a "large-scale, lower-cost, reproducible, and high-quality engineered process for broad industry and clinical use," Kotanchek said. The group is seeking to become a visionary and strategic international resource and an exemplar for developing new knowledge, innovative technologies, a diverse workforce, and enabling standards for the cell production and characterization processes.[1] The organization convenes critical stakeholders—including practitioners, industry professionals, regulators, and patient advocates—to address the necessary requirements for developing a lingua franca to facilitate communication among those working in biologics, informatics and analytics, and manufacturing and industrial engineering. CMaT is strategically positioned to address challenges in the emerging cell manufacturing industry, particularly those related to quality, cost, speed, and agility, she added. She focused on CMaT's work with multivariate critical quality attributes (CQAs), multivariate critical process parameters (CPPs), and how these influence the progress toward real-time monitoring.

---

[1] More information about CMaT is available at http://cellmanufacturingusa.org/vision (accessed January 8, 2021).

Dynamic Sampling Platform

Kotanchek described CMaT's dynamic sampling platform, which is designed to engineer reproducible, predictive measurement and assay technologies that enable batch and continuous monitoring of cell state and product. CMaT is working to develop nondestructive, in-line, closed system analysis using real-time sampling, reporters/sensors, and imaging tools as process analytic technologies. It is also developing three-dimensional disease and organoid models, also known as "potency-on-a-chip." The goal is to use this dynamic sampling platform in a robust way in both discovery and process development.

T Cell Characterization Project

The power of CMaT's approach, Kotanchek explained, lies in the recognition that key deliverables are needed in the formation of new scientific knowledge and in new tools and technologies that can be used to build integrated systems. Furthermore, CMaT recognizes that these building blocks can in turn be applied to different testbeds. She focused on an example specific to the T cell testbed. CMaT's work in this area links into its integrated, crosscutting engineering system, which is intended for use both for understanding the system and for predictive purposes, she added.

Kotanchek highlighted a project focused on variability in the assessment and omics characterization of CAR T cells through an integrative computational pipeline. This work explored how degradable microscaffold microcarrier cultures can expand more central memory and lymph-node-homing T cells (Dwarshuis et al., 2019). The goals of the project were to control these T cell expansion processes and to develop a workflow to enable multi-omics characterization and unbiased modeling of the end product for early, predictive signatures of quality during manufacturing. The project aims first to understand the variance and then to establish CQAs and CPPs that are predictive of potency, safety, and consistency.

The first phase of the project focused on examining the experimental process parameters by optimizing the microscaffold's input process parameters and looking at the responses of viability and CD4/CD8 naïve-memory attributes, Kotanchek said. The group employed DataModeler software, which uses evolutionary computing, to perform predictive optimization and identify regions for further improvement on extrapolation. Next, they executed a sequential, adaptive experimental design for further testing and validation, which enabled them to move into an optimized region that had not been part of the original study. Big data is often a focus of systems thinking, Kotanchek said, but much of their early program work actually involved smaller datasets and the use of the evolutionary toolset to gain a deeper understanding.

The second phase of the project—a multi-omics integrative approach for early predictive signatures—looked at the impact on microcarriers of process parameters, secretome profiles, and metabolites, Kotanchek said. This involved merging process parameters, secretomes, and nuclear magnetic resonance (NMR) data and measuring the total live CD4 naïve-memory cells, total live CD8 naïve-memory cells, and the ratios of CD4 to CD8. The objective was to examine if CD4 and CD8 cells could be controlled simultaneously, Kotanchek said, and this study also included a comparison of different machine learning analyses, along with linear modeling, to identify the best ways forward.

Determining the Modeling Options

When considering different algorithmic approaches, underlying assumptions are often overlooked, Kotanchek said. These underlying assumptions are generally tied to "what we believe we know and what we do not know." Specifically, they pertain to what is believed to be known about driving variables and about the model structure itself. For example, if the driving variables are known and the model form is linear, then linear regression may suffice. In cases where the driving variables are known and the model structure is nonlinear, then a nonlinear regression parameter may be appropriate. If the driving variables are known but the model structure is not, then a variety of powerful machine learning tools can be applied (e.g., neural networks, support vector machine model, random forests, and symbolic regression).

Symbolic regression can also be used in situations where there is uncertainty about the driving variables and of the model structure, Kotanchek said. This technique offers a powerful way to identify variables via the evolutionary process, providing explicit transparent models that can be tested. Evolution automatically handles the symbolic regression model development, generating novelty from the data that can then be exploited. Solutions are found by simulating natural evolutionary selection, with the end result being mathematical expressions instead of biological species. Novelty is generated by competition in the fitness of those expressions—in terms of accuracy versus complexity—to generate explicit algebraic, transparent, interpretable models. In this way, symbolic regression can be used as an augmented intelligence tool for hypothesis generation, enabling a domain expert to examine the most accurate solutions that emerge.

Learning and Extrapolating from Collections and Ensembles of Models

Not all models are created equal, Kotanchek noted, so the focus is on exploiting the collection of models that offer the greatest accuracy and the lowest degree of complexity. Focusing on the collection of models—rather than on specific models—can help to answer questions about: (1) modeling potential, (2) the complexity-versus-accuracy trade-off, (3) the number of variables required to get accurate models, (4) variable presence, (5) variable combinations, (6) variable and combination distributions, and (7) emergent metavariables that can provide further insight. The discussion of big data versus big insight is an important one in this type of work, Kotanchek said. The size of datasets can vary considerably—from 2 to 10,000 variables and from 10 to 1 million records—but the diversity of the dataset can be as important as its size; a dataset of 9 million records in which all but 10 are equivalent will not provide much insight into the early development process, for example, because it does not offer a diversity of data. It is critical to look at all data, she emphasized, including data that do not yield the anticipated result. The data themselves may help to determine the appropriate trade-off of complexity versus accuracy. Automated hypothesis generation and refinement serve to develop explicit algebraic models, reward simplicity and accuracy, and focus on the "good" and simple models. Many models are contenders, and all contenders can be exploited for insight and guidance. Iteration toward a final model set involves a focus on the variables that have the most impact on the outcome and on implementing a trustable model from the set of good and simple models.

A collection of models can be used to build "ensembles" of accurate-fit, trustable models. Ensembles are created by starting with interesting models that have reasonable accuracy and complexity, as well as desirable variables, variable combinations, and dimensionality. The models are automatically chosen to maximize the diversity of error residuals. Models within an ensemble will agree where constrained by data and diverge when exposed to novel parameter conditions. They can be used to guide decision making and to enable active learning and active design of experiments, Kotanchek added.

The diversity of the accurate-fit models in an ensemble is used to generate trust metrics, Kotanchek explained. To illustrate how ensembles are useful in extrapolation, she drew an analogy with the trajectory of a single bounce of a ball. If the simple trajectory is known and genetic programming were applied only to the first half of the bouncing ball dataset, it could generate hundreds of unique models to identify the prediction for the continued trajectory within seconds. A collection of simple models with high accuracy could then be selected to extract a diverse model set and generate an ensemble. This ensemble's trimmed mean provides a projection;

however, the space has not been fully exploited, so further information needs to be collected. If one took the same type of data and looked at other machine learning comparisons, they would not necessarily provide accurate projections.

The power of ensembles is in the active design of experiments through active learning, Kotanchek said. Using modeling, an ensemble can be generated that provides a projection for the trajectory. Even though the predicted trajectory would be inside the nominal data range, more data points are needed to proceed. By adding samples at the point of maximum divergence (i.e., along the top of the arc of the ball's bounce), it is possible to lock down model behavior, arriving at predicted trajectories that have little divergence from the actual trajectory. Thus, an active experiment design process can drive uncertainty out of the model. If experiments are expensive and time limited, Kotanchek added, ensembles can indicate areas where data collection will be most beneficial and informative. This concept of trustable models is the foundation of active experiment design, she emphasized.

Using Active Design of Experiments

CMaT has some key achievements that can be attributed to the active design of experiments, Kotanchek noted. These include optimizing conditions for maximizing memory T cells, designing the aforementioned CD4/CD8 multi-omics integration outputs, and designing the parameters for microcarriers and their interactive effects. CMaT has been able to merge the multi-omics dataset to run comparisons of accuracy and prediction across various machine learning methods (e.g., conditional inference forest, random forest, gradient boosted trees, and symbolic regression). These comparisons include all omics data, including data on process parameters over different time periods, process parameters with NMR, and process parameters with cytokine, Kotanchek said. The machine learning arm was performed to correlate and identify CPPs; it was effective in identifying cytokine dependency, examining the cytokines' interactive effect, and predicting total live memory, CD4, and CD8. In addition, CMaT used multi-omics prediction profiles based on NMR media analysis of ethanol and lactate and microcarrier characteristics to look at optimization. These processes can be performed simultaneously or independently if the objective is to optimize one versus the other, Kotanchek said.

Questions Driving the Systems Thinking Approach

When using a dynamic sampling platform, the issues to address include the identification of key factors, system design, and the potential for better solutions, Kotanchek said. A workflow approach can enable information to be extracted to inform the appropriate targets and designs for the dynamic platform. Active design of experiments is powerful, and system integration is paramount for the active learning process, she added. The active learning workflow integrates data sources, statistics and visualization, and data consolidation; this is followed by looking at model space descriptors, doing the modeling, deploying it through subject-matter experts, and then completing validation analysis. This information feeds back into the active design of the next set of experiments, and the cycle begins anew. She highlighted the importance of identifying the objective of the analysis at each phase of discovery, development, design, validation, optimization, process control, supply chain, commercialization, or strategy. This involves considering questions about variable selection and relationships, prediction, optimization and deployment, risk management, and insight and understanding (see Box 6-2). Kotanchek closed by encouraging researchers to exploit the data that are available, particularly experimental and manufacturing knowledge that relates to efforts that are not generating the target response. This type

---

BOX 6-2
Questions to Consider in Determining Analysis Objectives

Variable Selection and Relationships
- Which variables matter?
- What variable combinations are most useful?
- Are there important metavariables?

Prediction
- Can we accurately predict performance?
- What can we control in real time?

Optimization and Deployment
- Can robust emulators be built for what-if and design?
- Can we simultaneously optimize multiple key performance objectives?
- Can we build active learning systems?

Risk Management
- Can outliers be detected and assessed?
- What is the extrapolation trust metric?

Insight and Understanding
- Is it novel?
- Is it patentable?

SOURCE: Theresa Kotanchek workshop presentation, October 23, 2020.

of data can be powerful in understanding the difference between a patient group that is responding and a patient group that is not.

NOVEL SUPPLY CHAIN AND COST MODELING FOR CELL THERAPIES

Ben Wang, a professor, the executive director, and the Gwaltney Chair in Manufacturing Systems at the Georgia Tech Manufacturing Institute, discussed the application of systems thinking in manufacturing engineering, with a focus on novel supply chain and process modeling for regenerative medicine and cell therapy manufacturing and distribution. He presented several case studies of projects that have adopted a multidisciplinary approach to addressing the systems issue by building a team across different universities and disciplines. He also outlined two systems-based modeling projects and reviewed simulation case studies related to capacity planning, supply chain disruptions, demand surges and priority queue, and the cost of goods and automation.

Systems Thinking Lenses

Wang introduced three lenses through which to view systems thinking in manufacturing. The first is the technology readiness level/manufacturing readiness level spectrum, which moves through the stages of basic research, representative production environment, pilot product, low rate, full rate, and then finally the market. The second lens involves the value chain, whose stages include raw materials, fabrication, inspection, packaging, logistics, distribution, therapy delivery to patients, and long-term patient monitoring. The third lens is the stakeholders' view, in which systems are conceptualized as an ecosystem where all stakeholders work together in the effort to optimize a set of objectives. Not all objectives are aligned across various stakeholders, however, and objective optimizations can conflict in some cases, leading to potential dilemmas in decision making, Wang said.

Supply Chain Challenges in the Regenerative Medicine Ecosystem

To frame the use cases he presented, Wang provided an overview of how process modeling can be used to address supply chain challenges. Regenerative medicine supply ecosystems are complex, Wang said, and he highlighted three challenges in managing regenerative medicine supply chains (see Figure 6-1). First, the large variety of products and supply chain issues creates a system that involves both "push" and "pull" dynamics; interactions between the push and pull factors creates challenges. Next, in order to make regenerative medicine truly personalized, the health

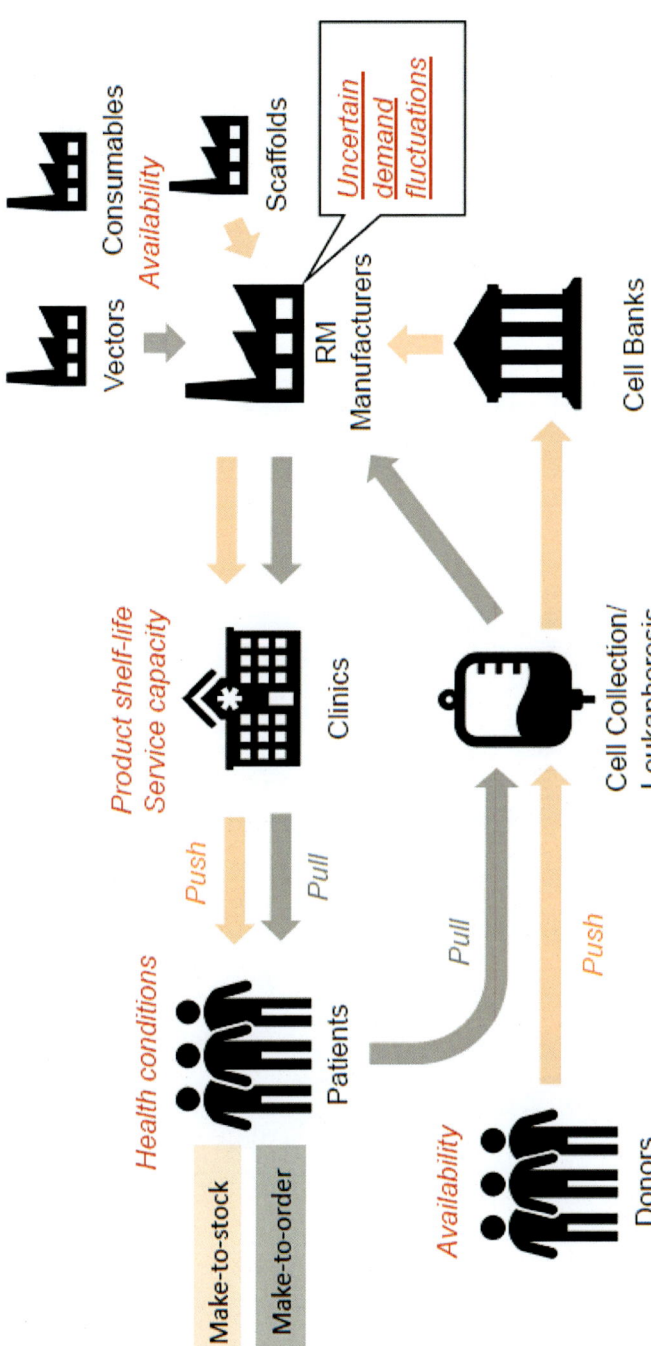

FIGURE 6-1 Complexity of regenerative medicine supply chain ecosystem.
NOTE: RM = regenerative medicine.
SOURCE: Ben Wang workshop presentation, October 23, 2020.

conditions of the patient must be considered throughout the entire process. This involves assessing the real-time impact of patient health conditions on production and supply chain planning and execution. The third challenge is that uncertainties abound, including uncertainties related to demand fluctuations, inevitable machine breakdowns, quality control and process failures, and supply chain disruptions.

Process Modeling to Address Supply Chain Challenges

Digital modeling has become an efficient and cost-effective approach to exploring the dynamics of the supply chain and the process models, Wang said. Many existing digital models focus on a narrow band of activities in the entire value chain, thus missing critical elements and tools (Lam et al., 2018). Wang described a supply chain and process modeling project designed to address this issue through four main objectives. The first is to build a decision-support toolset to incorporate all stakeholders' perspectives into supply chain system design, planning, and control. This involves attempting to optimize a set of stakeholder objectives that are not necessarily aligned and that may conflict. Second, the project aims to develop and validate digital models of manufacture and quality assurance for regenerative medicine and cells to support reliable, scalable manufacturing of quality, affordable therapeutics. These include models for a single production facility and for a network of production facilities. The third objective is to inform standards and the regulatory community in the process of standardizing this nascent industry. Finally, the project seeks to support and participate in education and workforce development, the importance of which cannot be overemphasized, Wang said.

The project adopted a two-pronged approach. The first prong is to develop a detailed view of a single production facility, such as a cell manufacturing facility or a regenerative medicine, tissue, or organ factory. Each component of the process is examined, from specimen collection to the point at which a therapy is packaged, inspected, and ready to be shipped. This involves assessing processing stations, quality control stations, human operators, and moving vehicles within the production facility. The second prong explores a network of facilities and generates various production model configurations. For example, a centralized production model would apply to a large factory being built in the United States to distribute products to clinics and hospitals throughout North America. A point-of-care production model would apply to a miniature production facility located at each hospital or clinic in the system. Configurations on the spectrum between centralized and point-of-care models uses the regional production hub model, which would apply to cases in which several factories are located throughout the country, each serving the hospitals and clinics within a corresponding region. These hubs may or may not interact with one another, reflecting the dynamic nature of this modeling, he added. Using digital modeling, the project has created models of both autologous CAR T cell manufacturing and allogeneic induced pluripotent stem (iPS) cell manufacturing, Wang said. It has developed simulation tools that provide decision makers with large amounts of information pertaining to production situations, use of resources, labor, lead times, quality, inventories, ordering status, and failure rates.

Use Case: Production Capacity Planning

Wang described a use case for production capacity planning. Capacity planning is of prime importance in a nascent industry such as regenerative medicine and cell manufacturing, he emphasized, where players do not have the decades of experience that players do in other industries, such as the aerospace and automotive industries. Capacity planning is critical for informing decisions such as the number of bioreactors to establish, the labor requirements needed, and the level of automation to consider over the next 5–15 years. Analytical and simulation tools can help decision makers and plant managers design the best configuration, he said.

Use Case: Supply Disruption Simulations

Wang presented another use case involving simulations on supply chain disruptions (e.g., a disruption in which a natural or humanmade disaster causes a major shortage in the production system of a key reagent). A simulation can be used to compare two production configurations. The first configuration is a simplified system comprised of one factory and one reagent supplier. The simulation predicted that a 60-day complete supply disruption would lead this lean production configuration to a substantial, lasting backlog, preventing any return to steady-state queue times. The second configuration contains one factory and two reagent suppliers. In this simulation, only one of the two suppliers is affected, while the other continues to operate. In this case, the facility would face a 50 percent supply disruption rather than a complete disruption. The result is shorter backlogs than in the first scenario and an eventual return to the original production steady state. Another simulation compared the configuration of one factory and one supplier with a configuration that included a second factory with its own supplier. In this example, a supply disruption affected the first factory's production, but the second factory and second supplier had no disruption. As in the preceding simulation, if the first factory halted production until the 60-day supply disruption ceased, the result would be a permanent backlog, with no return to steady state. In contrast, if the first factory were to transfer 50 percent of orders to the second factory, the resulting backlog would be time-limited, and eventually a return to steady state would be achieved. Thus, order transfer is one feasible risk-mitigation strategy, Wang said.

Use Case: Demand Surge Simulations

A more complicated simulation that Wang described involved responses to a significant demand surge. By comparing the impact of three risk-mitigation policies, it is possible to model demand surges of various intensities (e.g., 2- to 5-fold increases in demand of 20- to 60-day durations). The first risk-mitigation policy is to accelerate manufacturing, which might involve temporarily eliminating some of the final inspections in order to ship therapies more quickly to the sickest patients. The simulation revealed that this policy is useful for smaller demand surges and that the impact is independent of the duration of the surge. The second policy is a priority queue, in which the sickest patients are prioritized in cases where a surge causes wait time for therapy. This policy was found to be effective when the surge level is high, he said. The third policy is to combine accelerated manufacturing and priority queuing to employ mitigation strategies effective for both lower and higher surge levels, resulting in improvement across surge intensities and durations.

Use Case: Cost Modeling and Automation

Wang described a final use case that modeled automation for allogeneic iPS cell production and cost. Four different equipment configurations were compared: (1) a manual operation biosafety cabinet, (2) an automatic operation biosafety cabinet, (3) a manual operation isolator system, and (4) an automatic operation isolator system. Modeling revealed several takeaways. First, manual operations require much more labor, resulting in a lower throughput compared with automated systems. Also, isolators are more expensive and more labor intensive than biosafety cabinets. Finally, automation with biosafety cabinets has the lowest unit cost, whereas automation with isolators has the highest output. All of the configurations are assumed to be operating under the same cleanroom conditions, Wang said, but the factors of variability of cell quality and contamination risks have yet to be well studied.

DISCUSSION

Cell Quality in Manufacturing

How, Roy asked, could cell quality or CQAs influence the supply chain and automation system in the manufacturing pipeline? Cell quality and characterization or analytics were not considered in the model of automation cost and efficiency in Wang's final simulation example, he noted. Wang replied that from a manufacturing standpoint, standardization and simplification stages should take place before automation. First, he said, it is important to understand the process variables and CQAs as well as their relationship and interplays, which can simplify the process as much as possible. The second step is standardizing the process. It is a risky proposition to automate before the systems are standardized and most of the uncertainty has been removed, he cautioned.

Data Protection in Storage, Processing, and Sharing

What are some of the challenges associated with data storage, processing, and sharing, a workshop participant asked, particularly in translational settings when working with patient samples? This is a daily consideration in her work with Novartis, Tyagarajan said. Multiples sets of regulations are in place, including the Health Insurance Portability and Accountability Act, European Union regulations, and regional regulations. Furthermore, Novartis has internal regulations that must be met before looking at clinical trial data. After considering regulatory requirements, the company determines whether data can be stored in an environment that belongs to Novartis but is external to the location of the clinical trial data. When data are stored in this way, they are anonymized to remove as many patient identifiers as possible. In certain instances, Tyagarajan said, it is not possible to completely remove all patient-identifying data because linking between different databases can require preserving certain patient-identifying elements. In those cases, access to that particular column of data is controlled and limited to specific individuals. In such circumstances, calling for what are known as pseudonymized variables requires documentation that explains why these data cannot be completely anonymous. The company also conducts internal compliance checks to ensure that patient data are protected to the greatest extent possible. A sizable challenge in employing sophisticated machine learning approaches, Khalil added, is creating a method of aggregating and learning from data and feedback loops. This is particularly challenging for the manufacturing process in the context of the compliance required, she said.

Is there data sharing outside your company, Roy asked Tyagarajan, and do registries have a role to play with anonymized manufacturing data? Post-market chimera data are deposited in the Center for International Blood and Marrow Transplant Research database, he noted, but they do not include manufacturing and characterization data. Tyagarajan discussed several differences between registry data and clinical trial data which indicate that the latter are a much more complete dataset than registry data. Furthermore, as registries are not mandated in the United States, they are dependent on physicians' voluntary efforts to input information. Finally, patients may be less likely to report back to their physicians if they are doing well, contributing to incomplete data. An additional consideration relates to patient data acquired at different time intervals. For certain patients, data points may be collected at 6 months, 9 months, and 12 months. For others, it may be at 6 months and 12 months, and for still others it may be at 12 months and 24 months. Novartis has developed the pseudonymization process to help overcome this data gap. Partnerships and collaborations are needed, and this will require contracts and other formal steps, Tyagarajan said.

Registries have an important role to play, Khalil emphasized. While compliance can limit the data that can be shared, the AI Innovation Center advances patient care as much as possible within compliance. Registries can serve as a link between the manufacturing process and data on patient response over time. This type of registry can serve as a common platform where data modalities from those two pieces can be brought together, she said. With ongoing patient monitoring and the linkage of manufacturing with long-term patient outcomes, algorithms can be generated to provide the information that is most important for patients and doctors. However, she added, this will require collaboration among pharmaceutical companies, clinicians, and patient groups. The Multiple Myeloma Research Foundation has a registry on multiple myeloma patients followed longitudinally over time and, at this point, may even include data on novel cell therapies.[2] That registry has enabled advances in predicting disease progression and identifying patients' risk levels. These types of algorithms have benefits across the entire ecosystem, she concluded.

Discussions about accessing appropriate clinical data for these areas of research are ongoing, Kotanchek added. The next steps will involve (1) looking at long-term treatment effects, (2) integrating that knowledge with information from the manufacturing side in a way that allows the appropriate data to be shared, and (3) using the resulting deepened understanding to take additional action. She said that CMaT's efforts are potentially powerful but that access to clinical data in relation to those programs is

---

[2] More information on the Multiple Myeloma Research Foundation registry is available at https://mmrfcurecloud.org (accessed January 8, 2021).

essential. Thus, partnerships are paramount to realizing the full potential of what is possible.

Challenges Related to Lack of Patient Data

Are the types of patient data currently being collected (e.g., product characterization data, outcome data) sufficient, Roy asked, to predict treatment success? The lack of patient data in their clinical trials is a major challenge, Tyagarajan said. Her group uses the clinical trial dataset to train registry data, she said, but AI and machine learning require larger amounts of data. Because the field of cell and gene therapy is in its infancy, even the most advanced companies in the field have limited patient data. Thus, researchers often look to data collected by regional registries. These registries collect data from patients on a voluntary basis, and each has its own regulations. From a clinical outcome perspective, it is not possible to acquire the necessary amount of data from registries, but it is currently one of the only options available, Tyagarajan said.

In the chemical and biologics arena, situations with relatively low n and a high number of potential input variables are not uncommon, Kotanchek said. This has driven efforts to exploit the capability of symbolic regression to compress down to the highest probabilistic variables and variable combinations and then generate hypotheses. In contrast, more traditional machine learning tools are dependent on a very high n, which is used for feature identification. Symbolic regression capability allows for explicit inputs that can be checked by a domain expert to confirm that they make sense before they are used for building and testing. Therefore, the framework can be used to design the next set for validation, rather than waiting for the large n to arrive to drive those conclusions, she added.

The field of cell and gene therapy could learn from more mature industries that conduct process modeling for continuous improvement purposes, Roy said. Efforts are under way to structure informatics so that it can be reused across the enterprise to support various types of decision making, Kotanchek added. While confounding issues of patient data protection do present a substantial challenge, more investment is needed to support the reuse of data, she continued. Data assets are as critical as physical assets or human assets, yet they remain largely unexploited. New insights are valuable, Tyagarajan said, but they can create a time-consuming challenge. If a new insight pertains to a process that has already been validated, then it must be inputted into the regulatory filing. The philosophy of "process is product" may not apply to cell and gene therapy, Roy said. But if "the product is the product," then the process can vary to achieve that product. He suggested that the regulatory side of cell and gene therapy may need to evolve toward that mindset as well.

Availability of Simulation Tools

Are the evolutionary computing simulations that were discussed earlier in the session open source or proprietary? Kotanchek said that the results she shared came from a data modeler desktop tool available via licensed software, and evolutionary algorithms are also available. Open-source tools are not always the most efficient and do not always have constraints concerning overfitting, she said; this should be taken into account when choosing a tool. Sufficient algorithms are available in the public domain and in publications, Khalil added, but one challenge is the limited availability of experts in machine learning approaches who are actively working with clinical experts and experts in the manufacturing process to understand the fundamentals of the problem at hand. This expertise is needed to determine the appropriate underlying mathematics for those fundamentals. The uncertainty in a given ensemble should also be considered so that algorithms can be tailored to address that uncertainty. At that point, experts can develop methods to test the signals that are coming from the data. All of the components for that process already exist, Khalil said.

Facility Relocation Considerations

There are two sets of variables that companies must consider in relocation planning when thinking about optimization and modeling tools to assist companies looking to relocate a facility, Wang said. The first set is tangible and consists of configurations that can be based on the pros and cons of various generated models. The second set is less tangible and involves labor, skilled workforce, regulations, investment, infrastructure, and transportation. Roy asked how the supply chain fits into these variables. The initial investment (i.e., the capital expenditure) is a variable, Wang said. Long-term considerations involve variables related to cost, including labor, as well as logistics of storage, distribution, and access to ports, airports, and highway systems. This represents a different level of systems thinking, Roy commented. Moreover, while a company can enter a new market using an existing facility, relocating a facility is a huge hurdle, Tyagarajan said. Trained operators are the hardest commodity to obtain, but relocation is difficult without them. Timelines should be clearly established when planning a relocation, Tyagarajan said. The relocation process typically takes years, during which time the original process may have changed—and new knowledge acquired—that would need to be integrated into the facility, requiring another filing. The field of cell and gene therapy is moving much faster than the mammalian cell culture field, making it difficult to keep pace with the new technologies being developed and the associated commercial process that is filed. A process can become redundant by the time it is filed, Tyagarajan said, which creates another challenge.

Biological Information and Artificial Intelligence

Sui Huang, a professor at the Institute for Systems Biology, asked if biological knowledge—as mastered only by the human scientific mind—can be excluded from processes that rely on AI to extract actionable insights from big data or use automatic insights to determine causation. Our philosophy is to build biological measures into the process, Khalil said. This includes aspects such as cell viability, flow data from gene expression and omics, and process measures. She said that they take a probabilistic machine learning approach to the whole system. For example, the data may indicate that a key node, such as a certain genome, will drive cell count. Perhaps that genome was not measured in the first instantiation of the data. In this case, knowledge about how to account for hidden confounders or probabilistic models can be applied to capture the effect and then to inform collection of additional data. Khalil suggested that this is related to the issue of registries versus manufacturing because different types of data modalities can be combined to arrive at underlying biological mechanisms that are known to interact with process mechanisms.

7

Exploring Issues of Workforce Development Related to Systems Thinking

---

Important Points Highlighted by Individual Speakers

- With the emergence of systems thinking approaches in data science, artificial intelligence, and computational biology, individuals in the existing workforce may need to be re-trained or upskilled to interact with data in new modalities and interface across disciplines. (Balchunas)
- New strategies (e.g., providing support in managing student debt burdens, developing messaging to communicate the scientific importance and social impact of this work) are needed to recruit entrants into the workforce in the regenerative medicine and biopharmaceutical industries. (Gammie, Tilbury)
- Building teams of individuals with expertise in specific disciplines—who also have a foundational knowledge and competencies across multiple disciplines—can help develop a common language and provide a platform for collaborative innovation. (Tilbury, Zambon)
- Early and frequent engagement between industry and regulatory agencies can provide regulators with insight into cutting-edge work in the nascent field of cell and gene therapy as well as facilitating the coordination of industry-wide efforts to integrate systems thinking into drug development (Bollenbach, Tilbury, Zambon)
- Corporate leaders need to be educated about novel systems thinking approaches so that they can appreciate the overall value of new methodologies and understand the impact of these approaches on clinical trial and regulatory processes. (Bollenbach, Zambon)

The sixth workshop session featured a panel discussion which explored issues of workforce development related to systems thinking, with an aim of identifying challenges and opportunities for training and workforce development across fields such as data science, artificial intelligence (AI), and computational biology. The session was moderated by Tom Bollenbach, the chief technology officer at the Advanced Regenerative Manufacturing Institute. The session concluded with reflections on the workshop from the co-chairs.

EDUCATION AND WORKFORCE DEVELOPMENT TO ADVANCE SYSTEMS THINKING

Discussions about education and workforce development typically focus on the workforce deficit on the manufacturing and quality sides, Bollenbach said. However, there is also an acute need for a trained workforce that can operate in new analytical and data-rich environments. To develop the leaders of tomorrow, scientists and engineers should advocate for systems thinking approaches, Bollenbach said, and demonstrate the value of data-rich research and development in their places of work. Speaking from his manufacturing perspective, he shared his vision of a generation of scientists and engineers who "stop saying 'the process is the product' and start saying, '*this* process is the product, but we also know that these others are, too, because we have a robust understanding of and are well-informed by data.'"

Changing Workforce Development Needs

What are some of the most pressing challenges in workforce development, Bollenbach asked the panelists, particularly related to data science, AI, and computational biology? John Balchunas, the workforce director at the National Institute for Innovation in Manufacturing Biopharmaceuticals (NIIMBL), agreed that there is a need for additional manufacturing and quality talent. Although the fields of biopharmaceuticals and regenerative medicine are distinct, the workforce needs in these fields are similar, he said, and there are two challenges related to the changing workforce development needs that have been spurred by the proliferation of systems thinking. First, there is a need for re-training, or upskilling, the existing workforce so that they are able to interact with and respond to data, rather than routinely performing the same tasks each day. Given the interdisciplinary nature of this type of work, scientists should be able to interact with various stakeholders and operate in different modalities as needed, Balchunas said. Second, he continued, industries need to find ways to attract skilled, multidisciplinary talent. New approaches are needed to attract Ph.D.s, undergraduate students, and others to the fields of regenerative medicine and biopharmaceuticals—industries that are often in direct competition with large technology and software development companies that may appear more desirable for talented students preparing to enter the workforce.

Addressing Recruitment Challenges in the Field of Regenerative Medicine

Many talented students who would be well suited for work in the field of regenerative medicine are offered high-paying jobs in other industries even before completing their educational programs, said Alison Gammie, the director of training, workforce development, and diversity at the National Institutes of Health's (NIH's) National Institute of General Medical Sciences. The allure of a high-paying job is often strong, especially for students who have accumulated debt to pay for their education. Creative solutions should be developed to help workforce entrants manage their student debt burdens, she suggested. This issue also has a diversity dimension, she added, because underrepresented minorities carry a disproportionately high debt load (Addo et al., 2016).

Dawn Tilbury, the assistant director of engineering at the National Science Foundation (NSF), suggested that in addition to addressing the student debt load, it would be helpful to educate students in relevant areas of study about the importance of work being conducted in the regenerative medicine and biopharmaceutical fields. Students might be swayed if they realize that their contributions in these fields may have great social impact and may help save lives. The appeal of making an impact may offset the appeal of a high-paying job at a large technology firm. She added that students from underrepresented groups tend to have a greater affinity for jobs that have a tangible impact on people's lives. Manufacturing may have less allure than other technological fields, but it can offer workers high-impact, meaningful careers, Balchunas said. The industry should more clearly communicate this aspect of working in regenerative medicine, he added.

Training and Education Considerations in Workforce Development

Robert Zambon, the senior director of data strategy and external innovation at Johnson & Johnson, highlighted the need to recruit data scientists, analysts, and machine learning experts to the biopharmaceutical fields. Conversely, students in biology, chemistry, and other related scientific fields should be actively recruited into data science programs while still at university, if they show an interest. Students who study data science, AI, and machine learning tend to consider working either in the high-technology sector or in the biopharmaceutical industry—and view them as two distinct fields. Continuing to provide information about the different career options available to those who are currently in higher education—as well as those who are preparing to enter the workforce—would help to shift the balance and shape the workforce needed in the biopharmaceutical and regenerative medicine fields. Zambon also cautioned against focusing exclusively on trying to create polymaths who can do everything; instead, a better approach might be to focus on building teams in which different individuals have training in different areas of expertise.

Balchunas agreed that individuals need not be polymaths but said they should have a breadth of skills and competencies about the different disciplines they will act with in the field. The question, he said, is what foundational level of knowledge is needed for people working at the various levels within the biopharmaceutical and regenerative medicine industries. Providing a wide variety of skills and competencies as part of training may require a paradigm shift in the way the workforce is educated, he suggested. Tilbury drew an analogy with people who are able to speak not just their native tongue but other languages as well: students preparing to enter the workforce in these industries should be trained to speak a few words of the languages of other disciplines (e.g., chemistry, biology, data analytics, computer science) in order to remove the language barrier that can impede progress and collaborative problem solving in interdisciplinary fields. NSF is interested in exploring challenges related to interactions between disciplines to solve specific challenges, she added. In this type of "convergence research," multiple disciplines come together to learn each other's languages, tools, and data methods; this approach even offers the potential to create new disciplines. Bioinformatics, for example, is a relatively new discipline that emerged from the intersection of biology and information theory.

Promoting Interdisciplinary Competency

Are there ways, Bollenbach asked, to help biologists cultivate a greater appreciation and understanding of the physical sciences? Teams, Zambon suggested, should be built in a way that allows experts in different areas—such as an expert physicist and a biologist—to coordinate and work together toward respective goals that are similar, but not identical. When this type of collaboration is successful, the experts will often develop a common language through which they can understand each other's work, even if they are sometimes using the same term to represent completely different concepts in their respective disciplines. Developing these types of teams can bring together experts in data science, mathematics, computer science, biology, and genomics. Zambon described the result as a continuum; despite the variation in expertise and experience across this type of team, individuals start to come together naturally to fill gaps and build out new capabilities. In developing the workforce, he added, it is important to engage with undergraduate and graduate students to provide them with exposure to work in the field early on in their career development trajectories, for example, through fellowship programs and opportunities to rotate through different internal and external rotations. The strategy of bringing together a group of individuals with different areas of expertise to collaborate in an interdisciplinary project setting is relatively common in academic settings, Balchunas said. For instance, he runs a professional development program at the Biomanufacturing Training and Education Center at North Carolina State University[1] that assembles those studying engineering as well as different types of sciences at various levels to work together on specific projects. No matter what their educational background, the participants are learning all of the same content and taking the same approach, which, he said, has been effective in this program and at other universities with similar programs.

Bringing Systems Thinking to Regenerative Medicine Through the Workforce

How, Bollenbach asked, can industry and regulators help prepare the workforce to bring a systems thinking approach to regenerative medicine? From an industry perspective, Zambon replied, frequent engagement can help catalyze the move toward novel approaches and using data across the board in regenerative medicine. Regular networking can also help build relationships among various actors within regulatory agencies as new regulatory programs are instituted in different agencies. For instance, building relationships with regulators at the Food and Drug Administration (FDA) can ensure that they are familiar with the new products under development. FDA works extensively with various entities to help develop new plans and review activities on an ongoing basis, which can help identify routes to evolve. This provides regulatory agencies with insight into the field and helps coordinate industry-wide efforts. There could be a role for NSF engineering research centers and manufacturing innovation institutes (e.g., NIIMBL, BioFabUSA) to interact with FDA through a public–private partnership to transfer this knowledge, Bollenbach suggested. Tilbury agreed, emphasizing the importance of early engagement and partnership between industry and

---

[1]More information about the Biomanufacturing Training and Education Center at North Carolina State University is available at https://www.btec.ncsu.edu (accessed December 11, 2020).

regulatory bodies. Inviting representatives from regulatory agencies such as FDA and from manufacturing innovation institutes to participate in NSF's engineering research centers (ERCs) could be helpful, she suggested, so that they can follow research from its early stages to understand how the field will be moving forward. When NSF funds a phase I Small Business Innovation Research (SBIR) or Small Business Technology Transfer (STTR), FDA representatives are invited to the kickoff meeting with the researchers, which helps keep the regulatory environment in mind from the outset, she said.

Developing Roadmaps for Workforce Development

Asked whether there are training roadmaps being developed, Tilbury replied that some of NSF's ERCs develop curricula for students and training material for the next generation of the workforce. It would be helpful to engage with ERCs and other large centers that are simultaneously educating students and doing research to find out which types of skills they are seeking in their research students. NIIMBL has funded projects in education and workforce development that have developed curricula in areas such as data modeling, automation, and advanced analytics, Balchunas said. He said he was unaware of efforts to look specifically at workforce needs related to data analytics and systems, but he suggested that roadmaps developed for other industries could be adapted and applied. Gammie said that there are training programs available in this area. As a requirement of their NIH training grants, these programs are required to have specific, measurable goals in terms of students' outcomes and the skill set required to transition to the next level of the program. These programs are developed with a strong understanding of the career pathways available to the scientists they are training, which have overlap with a lot of the areas relevant to the workshop.

Bollenbach said that NSF recently funded an effort at the Georgia Institute of Technology[2] to develop a roadmap to look specifically at these education and workforce development challenges. This is important, he added, because while education and workforce development are very much a part of the work being done by BioFabUSA, NIIMBL, and the other manufacturing innovation institutes, their mandates are broad enough that they are often unable to dive in as deep as they would like on certain components, such as data science.

Janssen and Johnson & Johnson have established data science academies that focus not only on training and developing staff, but also on

---

[2] For more information on this NSF award to the Georgia Institute of Technology, see https://www.nsf.gov/awardsearch/showAward?AWD_ID=2036853&HistoricalAwards=false (accessed January 15, 2021).

educating executives, vice presidents, and corporate-suite officers about new capabilities, including systems thinking, that are emerging, Zambon said. Leadership also need to understand the common language and overall value of the new methodologies and approaches as they transition from the traditional approaches of past decades. Bollenbach agreed that members of leadership need to be educated about these novel approaches so that they can explain to investors why additional research and development is needed up front in product development to select sufficient and appropriate data prior to initiating clinical trials.

Strategies to Strengthen the Workforce

What steps can be taken within the next 3 years, Bollenbach asked, to strengthen and prepare the regenerative medicine workforce? There is a need for collaboration and synergies across various initiatives and stakeholders (e.g., NSF, BioFabUSA, NIIMBL, academia) to reduce the potential for redundancy by sharing ideas more broadly, Balchunas said. Tilbury suggested that the concept of "workforce" may be too vague. The concept encompasses Ph.D. students considering their career options, members of the existing workforce in need of new training, technicians, and others at different levels of the workforce with various types of expertise. She agreed with Balchunas's point about synergies, suggesting that there should be an inventory of what is currently happening in order to be able to identify specific gaps, needs, and opportunities in education and development for different cadres within the broader workforce. NSF would be willing to host a workshop to bring stakeholders together for such a discussion, she said. Zambon suggested raising awareness about how systems thinking, data science, analytics, AI, machine learning, and related fields affect people's everyday lives. Within the industry, internal data-science symposia could bring together an entire organization to show people the impact of data science, systems thinking, and other new approaches. These kinds of events can pique the interests of younger staff members and encourage them to seek training and find ways to integrate these new approaches into their own work on a day-to-day basis.

Bollenbach concluded the session by raising several open questions for future consideration. How do these topics affect broader workforce training? How should training in the regulatory science sector be carried out in order to take data science and systems thinking approaches into account? If AI is augmenting automation down the road, how will that affect the way quality control is done? In this case, quality control will not be carried out through chemistry, but rather by watching sensor data. How will validation be done, and will that change?

REFLECTIONS ON THE WORKSHOP

To close out the workshop, planning committee members Anne Plant, a National Institute of Standards and Technology (NIST) fellow and the former chief of NIST's Biosystems and Biomaterials Division, and Krishnendu Roy, the Robert A. Milton Chair Professor, the director of the NSF Engineering Research Center for Cell Manufacturing Technologies, and the director of the Marcus Center for Therapeutic Cell Characterization and Manufacturing at the Wallace H. Coulter Department of Biomedical Engineering at the Georgia Institute of Technology and Emory University, offered their reflections on what they had heard during the 2 days of presentations and discussion.

Theoretical Approaches to Large-Scale Data

The first session, Plant said, had focused on abstract ideas, theoretical models, and ways of thinking about data, information theory, landscape and gene network models, dynamic heterogeneity, and other high-level concepts. Access to large amounts of molecular-scale data does not guarantee the ability to predict what a biological system will do, she said; in addition, the data must be analyzed within an appropriate theoretical construct. Theoretical approaches for examining complex biological processes at the systems level largely involve assessing the probabilistic nature of biological outcomes and understanding how molecular components work together to produce the emergent biological characteristics of the system. The importance of emergent properties means that reliance on reductionist research approaches is no longer sufficient. It will be important to develop theoretical frameworks that help interpret the results of today's powerful omics tools and make it possible to understand how to use molecular data to predict emergent properties. Roy said that the discussion on potential landscapes and high probability attractor states suggests a guide for how to control manufacturing and differentiation processes. However, he said that realizing this promise of identifying the desirable cell population landscapes (e.g., the ideal cells to inject or use to make a tissue) will require integrating patient-level data into the systems-level analyses.

Challenges of Systems-Level Approaches

During the second session, Plant said, panelists converged on the ideas that a systems approach is critical for developing and manufacturing clinically successful products but that there are substantial challenges involved in implementing that approach. For instance, substantial resources will be needed to collect and analyze the volume of systems-scale data needed to identify emergent properties and develop new models.

Cross-Sector Collaborations for Developing and Sharing Datasets

The third session focused on how collaborative work across industry and academia through consortia can be applied to develop large data-sets—including real-world data—that can be analyzed using sophisticated methods, such as AI. Plant said that the presentations of examples of large-scale data-sharing efforts ongoing in the drug discovery and health care spaces demonstrate that it may be possible to achieve sufficient volume and scale of data to provide insight into complex patient profiles. These efforts suggest that data sharing at an even greater scale has the potential to provide a high-variable space in which to query patient response to complex products. Developing a common language, establishing cooperative strategies for collecting and sharing data, and making a strong business case for aggregating and sharing these large datasets could further facilitate coordinated efforts to identify major effects and emergent properties, which would in turn allow follow-up research on specific systems to identify specific targets. Plant noted that some presenters had indicated that regulators are increasingly interested and embedded in all of these activities. Roy added that patient data collected through consortia could be used to better understand how therapies affect patients at individual and group levels. Additionally, he said, active participation by regulators in this area will also be beneficial by reducing costs, reducing risks for industry, and accelerating product development.

Use of Data Modeling to Reduce Data Dimension to Key Variables

The fourth session explored the variety of model types and methods that can be applied within systems thinking approaches. A systems approach can help home in on those analytes and relationships that provide the most important predictive value, but identifying the most important contributors and their relationships requires analytical approaches that are designed to collapse state space. Plant said that these models go beyond simple cluster analysis by addressing matrix factorization in order to better understand how cell populations transition between phenotypes and by identifying cell dynamics, heterogeneity, and other characteristics. She added that there are significant modeling challenges to collapsing the molecular detail space to permit the identification of the major interactions that drive phenotype.

The fifth session, as Plant recounted, featured examples of how industry is using these types of systems-level modeling approaches, including a hierarchy of models to explore manufacturing processes. The negative consequences—both for patients and for industry—of failing to adopt a systems thinking approach in regenerative medicine were well established throughout the workshop, she said.

Cross-Disciplinary Training of the Workforce

The sixth session explored challenges related to recruiting talented students with computational skills into the regenerative medicine space when there are other lucrative career paths available to them. Plant highlighted the discussion around building teams containing a diversity of expertise rather than seeking out individuals who can "do everything."

FINAL WORDS ON MODELS AND DATA

The major challenges in applying systems thinking to regenerative medicine can be placed into two broad categories, Plant said: models and data. The field is still in the exploratory stage of building, improving, and evaluating models as well as developing a hierarchy of those models that can be used to explore the state of emergent properties. There are many modeling approaches, and each has pros and cons; for example, powerful machine learning models can be limited by the dearth of mechanistic information that they can provide. A major challenge related to data is the large size of the datasets required to conduct systems modeling in regenerative medicine. Obtaining these data at sufficient scale will require broad data-sharing efforts that protect both the privacy of patients and the intellectual property of industry. Additionally, real-world data that capture longitudinal measurements about long-term patient response need to be integrated with data on initial patient characteristics and manufacturing data (e.g., starting characteristics) in order to understand patients' outcomes over time.

Progress is being made toward systems thinking, Plant said, with modeling approaches that are less dependent on equations that describe the microscopic details of complex systems and models that focus on emergent or macroscopic phenomena, which might reveal the fundamental principles that guide how systems develop. For instance, using epigenetic landscapes to describe how cells transition to different states shows that biological outcomes can be framed as thermodynamic steady-state probabilistic processes related to stable attractor basins. These types of concepts can be used to understand complex systems in a more realistic way.

It is important to continue these types of interdisciplinary discussions that convene stakeholders from across the regenerative medicine field, Roy said. He proposed that the physics-based molecular modeling experts should engage with the machine learning, AI, and data-driven modeling communities to take advantage of the synergies between these disciplines in order to make better products and provide greater benefits to patients. Additionally, clinical trials should collect the right types of data in formats that are appropriate for use from the product side, the patient side, molecular side, and other elements of the ecosystem. Roy closed by highlighting the need for democratizing data and bringing more people "into the data umbrella" to develop innovative data-analytical tools that can be used to glean insights from research involving small sample sizes.

References

Abràmoff, M. D., P. T. Lavin, M. Birch, N. Shah, and J. C. Folk. 2018. Pivotal trial of an autonomous AI-based diagnostic system for detection of diabetic retinopathy in primary care offices. *npj Digital Medicine* 1(1):1–8.

Addo, F., J. N. Houle, and D. Simon. 2016. Young, black, and (still) in the red: Parental wealth, race, and student loan debt. *Race and Social Problems* 8(1):64–76.

Alberts, B., A. Johnson, J. Lewis, M. Raff, K. Roberts, and P. Walter. 2002. *Molecular biology of the cell, 4th edition*. New York: Garland Science; Drosophila and the Molecular Genetics of Pattern Formation: Genesis of the Body Plan. https://www.ncbi.nlm.nih.gov/books/NBK26906 (accessed May 14, 2021).

Altan-Bonnet, G., and R. N. Germain. 2005. Modeling T cell antigen discrimination based on feedback control of digital ERK responses. *PLOS Biology* 3(11):e356.

Altan-Bonnet, G., and R. Mukherjee. 2019. Cytokine-mediated communication: A quantitative appraisal of immune complexity. *Nature Reviews Immunology* 19(4):205–217.

Amigo, J. M., S. G. Balogh, and S. Hernandez. 2018. A brief review of generalized entropies. *Entropy (Basel)* 20(11):813.

Anderson, P. W. 1972. More is different. *Science* 177(4047):393–396.

Arnold, R. D., and J. P. Wade. 2015. A definition of systems thinking: A systems approach. *Procedia Computer Science* 44(2015):669–678.

Bachthaler, S., and D. Weiskopf. 2008. Continuous scatterplots. *IEEE Transactions on Visualization and Computer Graphics* 14(6):1428–1435.

Bargaje, R., K. Trachana, M. N. Shelton, C. S. McGinnis, J. X. Zhou, C. Chadick, S. Cook, C. Cavanaugh, S. Huang, and L. Hood. 2017. Cell population structure prior to bifurcation predicts efficiency of directed differentiation in human induced pluripotent cells. *Proceedings of the National Academy of Sciences* 114(9):2271–2276.

Beaupeux, M., and P. François. 2016. Positional information from oscillatory phase shifts: Insights from in silico evolution. *Physical Biology* 13(3):036009.

Bot, B. M., C. Suver, E. C. Neto, M. Kellen, A. Klein, C. Bare, M. Doerr, A. Pratap, J. Wilbanks, and E. R. Dorsey. 2016. The mPower study, Parkinson disease mobile data collected using ResearchKit. *Scientific Data* 3(1):1–9.

Burke, C. J., and C. Zylberberg. 2019. Sources of variability in manufacturing of cell therapeutics. *Regenerative Engineering and Translational Medicine* 5(4):332–340.

Caldwell, J., W. Wang, and P. W. Zandstra. 2015. Proportional-integral-derivative (PID) control of secreted factors for blood stem cell culture. *PLOS ONE* 10(9):e0137392.

Calude, C. S., and G. Longo. 2017. The deluge of spurious correlations in big data. *Foundations of Science* 22(3):595–612.

Chang, H. H., M. Hemberg, M. Barahona, D. E. Ingber, and S. Huang. 2008. Transcriptome-wide noise controls lineage choice in mammalian progenitor cells. *Nature* 453(7194):544–547.

Chen, X., S. Dallmeier-Tiessen, R. Dasler, S. Feger, P. Fokianos, J. B. Gonzalez, H. Hirvonsalo, D. Kousidis, A. Lavasa, and S. Mele. 2019. Open is not enough. *Nature Physics* 15(2):113–119.

Cherry, C., D. R. Maestas, J. Han, J. I. Andorko, P. Cahan, E. J. Fertig, L. X. Garmire, and J. H. Elisseeff. 2020. Intercellular signaling dynamics from a single cell atlas of the biomaterials response. *bioRxiv* 218537.

Clark, B. S., G. L. Stein-O'Brien, F. Shiau, G. H. Cannon, E. Davis-Marcisak, T. Sherman, C. P. Santiago, T. V. Hoang, F. Rajaii, and R. E. James-Esposito. 2019. Single-cell RNA-seq analysis of retinal development identifies NFI factors as regulating mitotic exit and late-born cell specification. *Neuron* 102(6):1111–1126.

Cohen, S., J. Roy, S. Lachance, J. S. Delisle, A. Marinier, L. Busque, D. C. Roy, F. Barabé, I. Ahmad, N. Bambace, L. Bernard, T. Kiss, P. Bouchard, P. Caudrelier, S. Landais, F. Larochelle, J. Chagraoui, B. Lehnertz, S. Corneau, E. Tomellini, J. J. A. van Kampen, J. J. Cornelissen, M. Dumont-Lagacé, M. Tanguay, Q. Li, S. Lemieux, P. W. Zandstra, and G. Sauvageau. 2020. Hematopoietic stem cell transplantation using single UM171-expanded cord blood: A single-arm, phase 1–2 safety and feasibility study. *Lancet Haematology* 7(2):e134–e145.

Csaszar, E., D. C. Kirouac, M. Yu, W. Wang, W. Qiao, M. P. Cooke, A. E. Boitano, C. Ito, and P. W. Zandstra. 2012. Rapid expansion of human hematopoietic stem cells by automated control of inhibitory feedback signaling. *Cell Stem Cell* 10(2):218–229.

Csaszar, E., K. Chen, J. Caldwell, W. Chan, and P. W. Zandstra. 2014. Real-time monitoring and control of soluble signaling factors enables enhanced progenitor cell outputs from human cord blood stem cell cultures. *Biotechnology and Bioengineering* 111(6):1258–1264.

Davis-Marcisak, E. F., T. D. Sherman, P. Orugunta, G. L. Stein-O'Brien, S. V. Puram, E. T. R. Torres, A. C. Hopkins, E. M. Jaffee, A. V. Favorov, and B. Afsari. 2019. Differential variation analysis enables detection of tumor heterogeneity using single-cell RNA-sequencing data. *Cancer Research* 79(19):5102–5112.

Deshpande, A., L.-F. Chu, R. Stewart, and A. Gitter. 2019. Network inference with Granger causality ensembles on single-cell transcriptomic data. *bioRxiv* 534834.

Dubuis, J. O., G. Tkačik, E. F. Wieschaus, T. Gregor, and W. Bialek. 2013. Positional information, in bits. *Proceedings of the National Academy of Sciences* 110(41):16301–16308.

Dwarshuis, N., H. W. Song, A. Patel, T. Kotanchek, and K. Roy. 2019. Functionalized microcarriers improve T cell manufacturing by facilitating migratory memory T cell production and increasing CD4/CD8 ratio. *bioRxiv* 646760.

FDA (Food and Drug Administration). 2018. *Advanced topics: Successful development of quality cell and gene therapy products.* PowerPoint slides available at https://www.fda.gov/media/80404/download (accessed February 10, 2021).

Ferrari, A., S. Lombardi, and A. Signoroni. 2017. Bacterial colony counting with convolutional neural networks in digital microbiology imaging. *Pattern Recognition* 61:629–640.

Fertig, E. J., J. Ding, A. V. Favorov, G. Parmigiani, and M. F. Ochs. 2010. CoGAPS: An R/C++ package to identify patterns and biological process activity in transcriptomic data. *Bioinformatics* 26(21):2792–2793.

Fertig, E. J., A. Markovic, L. V. Danilova, D. A. Gaykalova, L. Cope, C. H. Chung, M. F. Ochs, and J. A. Califano. 2013. Preferential activation of the hedgehog pathway by epigenetic modulations in HPV negative HNSCC identified with meta-pathway analysis. *PLOS ONE* 8(11):e78127.

Franco, R., and A. Cedazo-Minguez. 2014. Successful therapies for Alzheimer's disease: Why so many in animal models and none in humans? *Frontiers in Pharmacology* 5:146.

Goodfellow, I. J., Y. Bulatov, J. Ibarz, S. Arnoud, and V. Shet. 2013. Multi-digit number recognition from street view imagery using deep convolutional neural networks. *arXiv* 1312.6082.

Gordon, D. E., J. Hiatt, M. Bouhaddou, V. V. Rezelj, S. Ulferts, H. Braberg, A. S. Jureka, K. Obernier, J. Z. Guo, J. Batra, R. M. Kaake, A. R. Weckstein, T. W. Owens, M. Gupta, S. Pourmal, E. W. Titus, M. Cakir, M. Soucheray, M. McGregor, Z. Cakir, G. Jang, M. J. O'Meara, T. A. Tummino, Z. Zhang, H. Foussard, A. Rojc, Y. Zhou, D. Kuchenov, R. Hüttenhain, J. Xu, M. Eckhardt, D. L. Swaney, J. M. Fabius, M. Ummadi, B. Tutuncuoglu, U. Rathore, M. Modak, P. Haas, K. M. Haas, Z. Z. C. Naing, E. H. Pulido, Y. Shi, I. Barrio-Hernandez, D. Memon, E. Petsalaki, A. Dunham, M. C. Marrero, D. Burke, C. Koh, T. Vallet, J. A. Silvas, C. M. Azumaya, C. Billesbølle, A. F. Brilot, M. G. Campbell, A. Diallo, M. S. Dickinson, D. Diwanji, N. Herrera, N. Hoppe, H. T. Kratochvil, Y. Liu, G. E. Merz, M. Moritz, H. C. Nguyen, C. Nowotny, C. Puchades, A. N. Rizo, U. Schulze-Gahmen, A. M. Smith, M. Sun, I. D. Young, J. Zhao, D. Asarnow, J. Biel, A. Bowen, J. R. Braxton, J. Chen, C. M. Chio, U. S. Chio, I. Deshpande, L. Doan, B. Faust, S. Flores, M. Jin, K. Kim, V. L. Lam, F. Li, J. Li, Y. L. Li, Y. Li, X. Liu, M. Lo, K. E. Lopez, A. A. Melo, F. R. Moss, 3rd, P. Nguyen, J. Paulino, K. I. Pawar, J. K. Peters, T. H. Pospiech, Jr., M. Safari, S. Sangwan, K. Schaefer, P. V. Thomas, A. C. Thwin, R. Trenker, E. Tse, T. K. M. Tsui, F. Wang, N. Whitis, Z. Yu, K. Zhang, Y. Zhang, F. Zhou, D. Saltzberg, A. J. Hodder, A. S. Shun-Shion, D. M. Williams, K. M. White, R. Rosales, T. Kehrer, L. Miorin, E. Moreno, A. H. Patel, S. Rihn, M. M. Khalid, A. Vallejo-Gracia, P. Fozouni, C. R. Simoneau, T. L. Roth, D. Wu, M. A. Karim, M. Ghoussaini, I. Dunham, F. Berardi, S. Weigang, M. Chazal, J. Park, J. Logue, M. McGrath, S. Weston, R. Haupt, C. J. Hastie, M. Elliott, F. Brown, K. A. Burness, E. Reid, M. Dorward, C. Johnson, S. G. Wilkinson, A. Geyer, D. M. Giesel, C. Baillie, S. Raggett, H. Leech, R. Toth, N. Goodman, K. C. Keough, A. L. Lind, R. J. Klesh, K. R. Hemphill, J. Carlson-Stevermer, J. Oki, K. Holden, T. Maures, K. S. Pollard, A. Sali, D. A. Agard, Y. Cheng, J. S. Fraser, A. Frost, N. Jura, T. Kortemme, A. Manglik, D. R. Southworth, R. M. Stroud, D. R. Alessi, P. Davies, M. B. Frieman, T. Ideker, C. Abate, N. Jouvenet, G. Kochs, B. Shoichet, M. Ott, M. Palmarini, K. M. Shokat, A. García-Sastre, J. A. Rassen, R. Grosse, O. S. Rosenberg, K. A. Verba, C. F. Basler, M. Vignuzzi, A. A. Peden, P. Beltrao, and N. J. Krogan. 2020. Comparative host–coronavirus protein interaction networks reveal pan-viral disease mechanisms. *Science* 370(6521):eabe9403.

Gregor, T., D. W. Tank, E. F. Wieschaus, and W. Bialek. 2007. Probing the limits to positional information. *Cell* 130(1):153–164.

Guinney, J., and J. Saez-Rodriguez. 2018. Alternative models for sharing confidential biomedical data. *Nature Biotechnology* 36(5):391–392.

Gulshan, V., L. Peng, M. Coram, M. C. Stumpe, D. Wu, A. Narayanaswamy, S. Venugopalan, K. Widner, T. Madams, J. Cuadros, R. Kim, R. Raman, P. C. Nelson, J. L. Mega, and D. R. Webster. 2016. Development and validation of a deep learning algorithm for detection of diabetic retinopathy in retinal fundus photographs. *JAMA* 316(22):2402–2410.

Henry, A., M. Hemery, and P. François. 2018. Φ-evo: A program to evolve phenotypic models of biological networks. *PLOS Computational Biology* 14(6):e1006244.

Huang, S., G. Eichler, Y. Bar-Yam, and D. E. Ingber. 2005. Cell fates as high-dimensional attractor states of a complex gene regulatory network. *Physical Review Letters* 94(12):128701.

Kirouac, D. C., C. Ito, E. Csaszar, A. Roch, M. Yu, E. A. Sykes, G. D. Bader, and P. W. Zandstra. 2010. Dynamic interaction networks in a hierarchically organized tissue. *Molecular Systems Biology* 6:417.

Lam, C., E. Meinert, A. Alturkistani, A. R. Carter, J. Karp, A. Yang, D. Brindley, and Z. Cui. 2018. Decision support tools for regenerative medicine: Systematic review. *Journal of Medical Internet Research* 20(12):e12448.

Laughlin, S. 1981. A simple coding procedure enhances a neuron's information capacity. *Zeitschrift für Naturforsch C* 36(9–10):910–912.

Lim, H., and H. Shin. 2013. Classification and Characteristics of Fed-Batch Cultures. In *Fed-Batch cultures: Principles and applications of semi-batch bioreactors* (Cambridge Series in Chemical Engineering, pp. 62–84). Cambridge, UK: Cambridge University Press.

Lipniacki, T., B. Hat, J. R. Faeder, and W. S. Hlavacek. 2008. Stochastic effects and bistability in T cell receptor signaling. *Journal of Theoretical Biology* 254(1):110–122.

Lipsitz, Y. Y., N. E. Timmins, and P. W. Zandstra. 2016. Quality cell therapy manufacturing by design. *Nature Biotechnology* 34(4):393–400.

Liu, X., Y. Chen, J. Bae, H. Li, J. Johnston, and T. Sanger. 2019. *Predicting heart failure readmission from clinical notes using deep learning.* Paper read at 2019 IEEE International Conference on Bioinformatics and Biomedicine (BIBM), November 18–21. https://arxiv.org/abs/1912.10306 (accessed March 22, 2021).

Ly, T., C. Pamer, O. Dang, S. Brajovic, S. Haider, T. Botsis, D. Milward, A. Winter, S. Lu, and R. Ball. 2018. Evaluation of natural language processing (NLP) systems to annotate drug product labeling with MedDRA terminology. *Journal of Biomedical Informatics* 83:73–86.

Manyika. J., M. Chui, B. Brown, J. Bughin, R. Dobbs, C. Roxburgh, and A. H. Byers. 2011. Big data: The next frontier for innovation, competition, and productivity. New York: McKinsey Global Institute. https://www.mckinsey.com/business-functions/mckinsey-digital/our-insights/big-data-the-next-frontier-for-innovation (accessed January 13, 2021).

Melsted, P., A. S. Booeshaghi, F. Gao, E. da Veiga Beltrame, L. Lu, K. E. Hjorleifsson, J. Gehring, and L. Pachter. 2019. Modular and efficient pre-processing of single-cell RNA-seq. *bioRxiv* 673285.

Mojtahedi, M., A. Skupin, J. Zhou, I. G. Castaño, R. Y. Leong-Quong, H. Chang, K. Trachana, A. Giuliani, and S. Huang. 2016. Cell fate decision as high-dimensional critical state transition. *PLOS Biology* 14(12):e2000640.

Mueller, K. T., E. Waldron, S. A. Grupp, J. E. Levine, T. W. Laetsch, M. A. Pulsipher, M. W. Boyer, K. J. August, J. Hamilton, and R. Awasthi. 2018. Clinical pharmacology of tisagenlecleucel in B-cell acute lymphoblastic leukemia. *Clinical Cancer Research* 24(24):6175–6184.

NASEM (National Academies of Sciences, Engineering, and Medicine). 2017. *Navigating the manufacturing process and ensuring the quality of regenerative medicine therapies: Proceedings of a workshop.* Washington, DC: The National Academies Press.

NCMC (National Cell Manufacturing Consortium). 2016. Achieving large-scale, cost-effective, reproducible manufacturing of high-quality cells: A technology roadmap to 2025. http://www.cellmanufacturingusa.org/sites/default/files/NCMC_Roadmap_021816_high_res-2.pdf (accessed January 6, 2021).

Neelapu, S. S., F. L. Locke, N. L. Bartlett, L. J. Lekakis, D. B. Miklos, C. A. Jacobson, I. Braunschweig, O. O. Oluwole, T. Siddiqi, and Y. Lin. 2017. Axicabtagene ciloleucel CAR T cell therapy in refractory large B-cell lymphoma. *New England Journal of Medicine* 377(26):2531–2544.

Nielsen, M. 2015. *Neural networks and deep learning.* Determination Press. Online book. http://neuralnetworksanddeeplearning.com (accessed January 24, 2021).

REFERENCES

Opdam, S., A. Richelle, B. Kellman, S. Li, D. C. Zielinski, and N. E. Lewis. 2017. A systematic evaluation of methods for tailoring genome-scale metabolic models. *Cell Systems* 4(3):318–329.

Palpant, N. J., P. Hofsteen, L. Pabon, H. Reinecke, and C. E. Murry. 2015. Cardiac development in zebrafish and human embryonic stem cells is inhibited by exposure to tobacco cigarettes and e-cigarettes. *PLOS ONE* 10(5):e0126259.

Petkova, M. D., G. Tka ik, W. Bialek, E. F. Wieschaus, and T. Gregor. 2019. Optimal decoding of cellular identities in a genetic network. *Cell* 176(4):844–855.

Poplin, R., A. V. Varadarajan, K. Blumer, Y. Liu, M. V. McConnell, G. S. Corrado, L. Peng, and D. R. Webster. 2018. Prediction of cardiovascular risk factors from retinal fundus photographs via deep learning. *Nature Biomedical Engineering* 2(3):158–164.

Proulx-Giraldeau, F., T. J. Rademaker, and P. François. 2017. Untangling the hairball: Fitness-based asymptotic reduction of biological networks. *Biophysical Journal* 113(8):1893–1906.

Pulla, P. 2019. The plan to mine the world's research papers. *Nature* 571(7766):316–319.

Qiao, W., W. Wang, E. Laurenti, A. L. Turinsky, S. J. Wodak, G. D. Bader, J. E. Dick, and P. W. Zandstra. 2014. Intercellular network structure and regulatory motifs in the human hematopoietic system. *Molecular Systems Biology* 10(7):741.

Ray, S., and S. Pyne. 2012. A computational framework to emulate the human perspective in flow cytometric data analysis. *PLOS ONE* 7(5):e35693.

Richelle, A., and M. van Stosch. 2020. From big data to precise understanding: The quest for meaningful information. *Bio Process International*, February 6. https://bioprocessintl.com/manufacturing/information-technology/systems-biology-tools-for-big-data-in-the-biopharmaceutical-industry (accessed January 13, 2021).

Richelle, A., B. David, D. Demaegd, M. Dewerchin, R. Kinet, A. Morreale, R. Portela, Q. Zune, and M. von Stosch. 2020. Towards a widespread adoption of metabolic modeling tools in biopharmaceutical industry: A process systems biology engineering perspective. *npj Systems Biology and Applications* 6(1):6.

Riley, P. 2019. Three pitfalls to avoid in machine learning. *Nature* 572:27–29.

Rudrapatna, V. A., and A. J. Butte. 2020. Opportunities and challenges in using real-world data for health care. *Journal of Clinical Investigation* 130(2):565–574.

Schadt, E. E., J. Lamb, X. Yang, J. Zhu, S. Edwards, D. GuhaThakurta, S. K. Sieberts, S. Monks, M. Reitman, and C. Zhang. 2005. An integrative genomics approach to infer causal associations between gene expression and disease. *Nature Genetics* 37(7):710–717.

Sieberts, S. K., J. Schaff, M. Duda, B. Á. Pataki, M. Sun, P. Snyder, J. F. Daneault, F. Parisi, G. Costante, U. Rubin, P. Banda, Y. Chae, E. Chaibub Neto, E. R. Dorsey, Z. Aydın, A. Chen, L. L. Elo, C. Espino, E. Glaab, E. Goan, F. N. Golabchi, Y. Görmez, M. K. Jaakkola, J. Jonnagaddala, R. Klén, D. Li, C. McDaniel, D. Perrin, T. M. Perumal, N. M. Rad, E. Rainaldi, S. Sapienza, P. Schwab, N. Shokhirev, M. S. Venäläinen, G. Vergara-Diaz, Y. Zhang, Parkinson's Disease Digital Biomarker Challenge Consortium, Y. Wang, Y. Guan, D. Brunner, P. Bonato, L. M. Mangravite, and L. Omberg. 2021. Crowdsourcing digital health measures to predict Parkinson's disease severity: The Parkinson's disease digital biomarker DREAM Challenge. *NPJ Digital Medicine* 4(1):53.

Stein-O'Brien, G. L., R. Arora, A. C. Culhane, A. V. Favorov, L. X. Garmire, C. S. Greene, L. A. Goff, Y. Li, A. Ngom, and M. F. Ochs. 2018. Enter the matrix: Factorization uncovers knowledge from omics. *Trends in Genetics* 34(10):790–805.

Stein-O'Brien, G. L., B. S. Clark, T. Sherman, C. Zibetti, Q. Hu, R. Sealfon, S. Liu, J. Qian, C. Colantuoni, and S. Blackshaw. 2019. Decomposing cell identity for transfer learning across cellular measurements, platforms, tissues, and species. *Cell Systems* 8(5):395–411.

Tewary, M., N. Shakiba, and P. W. Zandstra. 2018. Stem cell bioengineering: Building from stem cell biology. *Nature Reviews Genetics* 19(10):595–614.

Till, J. E., E. A. McCulloch, and L. Siminovitch. 1964. A stochastic model of stem cell proliferation, based on the growth of spleen colony-forming cells. *Proceedings of the National Academy of Sciences* 51(1):29–36.

Tkačik, G., C. G. Callan, and W. Bialek. 2008. Information flow and optimization in transcriptional regulation. *Proceedings of the National Academy of Sciences* 105(34):12265–12270.

Topol, E. J. 2019. High-performance medicine: The convergence of human and artificial intelligence. *Nature Medicine* 25:44–56.

Trachana, K., R. Bargaje, G. Glusman, N. D. Price, S. Huang, and L. E. Hood. 2018. Taking systems medicine to heart. *Circulation Research* 122(9):1276–1289.

Trapnell C., D. Cacchiarelli, J. Grimsby, P. Pokharel, S. Li, M. Morse, N. J. Lennon, K. J. Livak, T. S. Mikkelsen, and J. L. Rinn. 2014. The dynamics and regulators of cell fate decisions are revealed by pseudotemporal ordering of single cells. *Nature Biotechnology* 32(4):381–386.

Tsokas, K., R. McFarland, C. Burke, J. L. Lynch, T. Bollenbach, D. A. Callaway II, and J. Siegel. 2019. Reducing risks and delays in the translation of cell and gene therapy innovations into regulated products. *NAM Perspectives*. Discussion paper. Washington, DC: The National Academies Press.

Turing, A. M. 1952. The chemical basis of morphogenesis. *Bulletin of Mathematical Biology* 52(1–2):153–197.

Verhoeff, R. P., M.-C. P. Knippels, M. G. Gilissen, and K. T. Boersma. 2018. The theoretical nature of systems thinking. Perspectives on systems thinking in biology education. *Frontiers in Education.* https://doi.org/10.3389/feduc.2018.00040.

Waddington, C. H. 1957. *The strategy of the genes*. New York: Routledge.

Wagner, A., A. Regev, and N. Yosef. 2016. Revealing the vectors of cellular identity with single-cell genomics. *Nature Biotechnology* 34(11):1145–1160.

Wan, Y.-W., R. Al-Ouran, C. G. Mangleburg, T. M. Perumal, T. V. Lee, K. Allison, V. Swarup, C. C. Funk, C. Gaiteri, M. Allen, M. Wang, S. M. Neuner, C. C. Kaczorowski, V. M. Philip, G. R. Howell, H. Martini-Stoica, H. Zheng, H. Mei, X. Zhong, J. W. Kim, V. L. Dawson, T. M. Dawson, P.-C. Pao, L.-H. Tsai, J.-V. Haure-Mirande, M. E. Ehrlich, P. Chakrabarty, Y. Levites, X. Wang, E. B. Dammer, G. Srivastava, S. Mukherjee, S. K. Sieberts, L.Omberg, K. D. Dang, J. A. Eddy, P. Snyder, Y. Chae, S. Amberkar, W. Wei, W. Hide, C. Preuss, A. Ergun, P. J. Ebert, D. C. Airey, S. Mostafavi, L. Yu, H.-U. Klein, Accelerating Medicines Partnership–Alzheimer's Disease Consortium, G. W. Carter, D. A. Collier, T. E. Golde, A. I. Levey, D. A. Bennett, K. Estrada, T. M. Townsend, B. Zhang, E. Schadt, P. L. De Jager, N. D. Price, N. Ertekin-Taner, Z. Liu, J. M. Shulman, L. M. Mangravite, and B. A. Logsdon. 2020. Meta-analysis of the Alzheimer's disease human brain transcriptome and functional dissection in mouse models. *Cell Reports* 32(2):107908.

Way, G. P., M. Zietz, V. Rubinetti, D. S. Himmelstein, and C. S. Greene. 2020. Compressing gene expression data using multiple latent space dimensionalities learns complementary biological representations. *Genome Biology* 21:109.

Wu, L., D. Wang, and J. A. Evans. 2019. Large teams develop and small teams disrupt science and technology. *Nature* 566(7744):378–382.

Wuchty, S., B. F. Jones, and B. Uzzi. 2007. The increasing dominance of teams in production of knowledge. *Science* 316(5827):1036–1039.

Xue, Q., E. Bettini, P. Paczkowski, C. Ng, A. Kaiser, T. McConnell, O. Kodrasi, M. F. Quigley, J. Heath, and R. Fan. 2017. Single-cell multiplexed cytokine profiling of CD19 CAR-T cells reveals a diverse landscape of polyfunctional antigen-specific response. *Journal for Immunotherapy of Cancer* 5(1):85.

Zhou, J. X., M. Aliyu, E. Aurell, and S. Huang. 2012. Quasi-potential landscape in complex multi-stable systems. *Journal of the Royal Society Interface* 9(77):3539–3553.

Appendix A

Workshop Agenda

Applying Systems Thinking to Regenerative Medicine: A Workshop

October 22–23, 2020
Virtual Workshop

TIMELINE:
October 22: 11:00 a.m.–4:00 p.m. ET
October 23: 10:00 a.m.–2:00 p.m. ET

DAY 1: October 22, 2020

11:00 a.m. ET   **Welcome from the Forum Co-Chairs**
TIM COETZEE, *Forum Co-Chair*
Chief Advocacy, Services, and Research Officer
National Multiple Sclerosis Society

KATHY TSOKAS, *Forum Co-Chair*
Regulatory Head of Regenerative Medicine &
    Advanced Therapy
Johnson & Johnson

11:10 a.m. **Introduction and Charge to the Workshop Speakers and Participants**
ANNE PLANT, *Workshop Planning Committee Co-Chair*
Fellow, National Institute of Standards and Technology

KRISHNENDU ROY, *Workshop Planning Committee Co-Chair*
Robert A. Milton Chair Professor
Director, Engineering Research Center for Cell Manufacturing Technologies
National Science Foundation Engineering Research Center for Cell Manufacturing Technologies
Director, Marcus Center for Therapeutic Cell Characterization and Manufacturing, Wallace H. Coulter Department of Biomedical Engineering
Georgia Institute of Technology and Emory University

SESSION I: INTRODUCTION TO SYSTEMS THINKING CONCEPTS

Moderator: Claudia Zylberberg, Akron Biotech

Session Objectives:
- Provide important background and an introduction to systems thinking approaches and related terminology.
- Explore specific examples of how systems thinking has been applied to areas of health and medicine, including potential opportunities in the regenerative medicine space.

11:20 a.m. **An Introduction to Systems Thinking**
WILLIAM BIALEK
John Archibald Wheeler/Battelle Professor in Physics, Lewis-Sigler Institute for Integrative Genomics
Princeton University

11:35 a.m.	**Applying Systems Thinking to the Development of Regenerative Medicines** PETER ZANDSTRA Director, Michael Smith Laboratories Director and Professor, School of Biomedical Engineering The University of British Columbia
11:50 a.m.	**Computational Approaches for Systems-Level Data Collection** SUI HUANG Professor Institute for Systems Biology
12:05 p.m.	**Q&A with the Speakers and Participants**
12:30 p.m.	**Break**

SESSION II: THE CHALLENGE OF CRITICAL QUALITY ATTRIBUTES: THE ROLE OF SYSTEMS THINKING

Moderator: Anne Plant, National Institute of Standards and Technology

Session Objective:
- Understand the challenges associated with identifying critical quality attributes in the discovery, regulation, and manufacturing of regenerative medicine products and how systems thinking approaches may be applied.

1:00 p.m.	**Fireside Chat: Systems Thinking and the Regulation of Regenerative Medicine Products** AMY ABERNETHY Principal Deputy Commissioner of Food and Drugs Food and Drug Administration
1:15 p.m.	**Q&A with the Audience**
1:30 p.m.	**Costs Associated with *Not Implementing* Systems Thinking Approaches—A Panel Discussion** *Moderator:* JANE LEBKOWSKI President Regenerative Patch Technologies

Panelists:
ADRIAN BOT
Vice President and Global Head, Translational
 Medicine
Kite Pharma, Inc.

BALA MANIAN
Chief Executive Officer
Mojave Bio, Inc.

DOUGLAS OLSON
President and Chief Executive Officer,
 BUHLMANN Diagnostics Corp.
Scientific Advisory Board Member, Cell Manufacturing
 Technologies

SALLY TEMPLE
Scientific Director, Principal Investigator, and
 Co-Founder
Neural Stem Cell Institute

2:15 p.m.   **Break**

SESSION III: CHALLENGES ASSOCIATED WITH DATA COLLECTION, AGGREGATION, AND SHARING

Moderator: Sadik Kassim, Vor Biopharma

Session Objectives:
- Discuss how big data can be leveraged to identify which patients will respond best to a particular regenerative medicine.
- Highlight challenges in data collection and data sharing such as small sample size in clinical trials, proprietary issues, and patient privacy.

2:45 p.m.   **Data Challenges with Omics Analysis and Disease Modeling**
LARSSON OMBERG
Vice President, Systems Biology
Sage Bionetworks

APPENDIX A   *131*

3:00 p.m.	**Using Big Data for Clinical Stratification of Patients** ATUL BUTTE Priscilla Chan and Mark Zuckerberg Distinguished Professor Director, Bakar Computational Health Sciences Institute University of California, San Francisco
3:15 p.m.	**Moderated Panel Discussion**
3:45 p.m.	**Reflections on Day 1 and Preview of Day 2** ANNE PLANT, *Workshop Planning Committee Co-Chair* Fellow, National Institute of Standards and Technology KRISHNENDU ROY, *Workshop Planning Committee Co-Chair* Robert A. Milton Chair Professor Director, Engineering Research Center for Cell Manufacturing Technologies National Science Foundation Engineering Research Center for Cell Manufacturing Technologies Director, Marcus Center for Therapeutic Cell Characterization and Manufacturing, Wallace H. Coulter Department of Biomedical Engineering Georgia Institute of Technology and Emory University
4:00 p.m.	**Adjourn Workshop Day 1**

DAY 2: October 23, 2020

10:00 a.m. ET	**Welcome and Overview of Day 2** ANNE PLANT, *Workshop Planning Committee Co-Chair* Fellow, National Institute of Standards and Technology

KRISHNENDU ROY, *Workshop Planning Committee Co-Chair*
Robert A. Milton Chair Professor
Director, Engineering Research Center for Cell Manufacturing Technologies
National Science Foundation Engineering Research Center for Cell Manufacturing Technologies
Director, Marcus Center for Therapeutic Cell Characterization and Manufacturing, Wallace H. Coulter Department of Biomedical Engineering
Georgia Institute of Technology and Emory University

SESSION IV: CHALLENGES AND OPPORTUNITIES ASSOCIATED WITH SYSTEMS-LEVEL ANALYSIS AND MODELING

Moderator: Malcolm Moos, Food and Drug Administration

Session Objectives:
- Discuss the current state of the art of systems thinking approaches and how these approaches are being used to inform identification of important variables to measure.
- Illuminate current gaps in knowledge and areas for further study.

10:10 a.m.	**Developing Algorithms for Single-Cell Genomics** ELANA FERTIG Associate Professor, Oncology Johns Hopkins University
10:25 a.m.	**Adopting Metabolic Modeling Tools in the Biopharmaceutical Industry** ANNE RICHELLE Senior Specialist, Metabolic Modeling GlaxoSmithKline
10:40 a.m.	**Modeling Dynamic Data to Identify a Reduced Variable Space** PAUL FRANCOIS Associate Professor, Department of Physics McGill University
10:55 a.m.	**Moderated Panel Discussion**
11:15 a.m.	**Break**

SESSION V: ADDRESSING REGENERATIVE MEDICINE MANUFACTURING AND SUPPLY CHAIN CHALLENGES WITH SYSTEMS-LEVEL APPROACHES

Moderator: Krishnendu Roy, Georgia Institute of Technology

Session Objective:
- Highlight opportunities where systems thinking approaches could address inefficiencies with manufacturing and the supply chain related to regenerative medicine.

11:45 a.m.	**Overview of Artificial Intelligence in Cell and Gene Therapies** IYA KHALIL Global Head of the AI Innovation Center Novartis SESHU TYAGARAJAN Global Head, Late-Stage Chemistry, Manufacturing, and Control Strategy Novartis
12:00 p.m.	**Modeling the Manufacturing Process in Regenerative Medicine** THERESA KOTANCHEK Chief Executive Officer Evolved Analytics, LLC
12:15 p.m.	**Supply Chain and Cost Modeling** BEN WANG Gwaltney Chair in Manufacturing Systems Professor and Executive Director Georgia Tech Manufacturing Institute
12:30 p.m.	**Moderated Panel Discussion**
1:00 p.m.	**Break**

SESSION VI: EXPLORING ISSUES OF WORKFORCE DEVELOPMENT RELATED TO SYSTEMS THINKING

1:20 p.m. Challenges and Opportunities for Training and Workforce Development in Data Science, Artificial Intelligence, and Computational Biology: A Panel Discussion

Moderator:
TOM BOLLENBACH
Chief Technology Officer
Advanced Regenerative Manufacturing Institute

Panelists:
JOHN BALCHUNAS
Workforce Director
The National Institute for Innovation in Manufacturing Biopharmaceuticals

ALISON GAMMIE
Director of Training, Workforce Development and Diversity
National Institute of General Medical Sciences
National Institutes of Health

DAWN TILBURY
Assistant Director, Engineering
National Science Foundation

ROBERT ZAMBON
Senior Director, Data Strategy and External Innovation
Johnson & Johnson

1:50 p.m. **Reflections from the Workshop and Final Comments**
ANNE PLANT, *Workshop Planning Committee Co-Chair*
Fellow, National Institute of Standards and Technology

KRISHNENDU ROY, *Workshop Planning Committee Co-Chair*
Robert A. Milton Chair Professor
Director, Engineering Research Center for Cell Manufacturing Technologies
National Science Foundation Engineering Research Center for Cell Manufacturing Technologies
Director, Marcus Center for Therapeutic Cell Characterization and Manufacturing, Wallace H. Coulter Department of Biomedical Engineering
Georgia Institute of Technology and Emory University

2:00 p.m. **Adjourn Workshop Day 2**

Appendix B

Speaker Biographical Sketches

Amy Abernethy, M.D., is the principal deputy commissioner of food and drugs at the Food and Drug Administration (FDA) and helps oversee the agency's day-to-day functioning and directs special and high-priority initiatives that cut across offices overseeing FDA's regulation of drugs, medical devices, tobacco, and food. As the acting chief information officer, she oversees FDA's data and technical vision and its execution. Dr. Abernethy, a hematologist/oncologist and palliative medicine physician, is an internationally recognized clinical data expert and clinical researcher. Her areas of expertise include cancer data, real-world evidence, clinical trials, health services research, patient-reported outcomes, clinical informatics, and patient-centered care. Before coming to FDA, Dr. Abernethy served as the chief medical officer, the chief scientific officer, and the senior vice president for oncology at Flatiron Health (a member of the Roche Group), where she led the research oncology, clinical operations, and data science teams and contributed to the overall strategic vision of the company, including directing its research vision on real-world evidence. Prior to that, Dr. Abernethy was a professor of medicine at the Duke University School of Medicine, where she ran the Center for Learning Health Care in the Duke Clinical Research Institute and the Duke Cancer Care Research Program in the Duke Cancer Institute. At Duke, she pioneered the development of technology platforms to spur novel advances in the care of people with cancer and other serious life-limiting illnesses. Dr. Abernethy was formerly an appointed member of the National Academies of Sciences, Engineering, and Medicine's National Cancer Policy Forum, an elected member of the American Society for Clinical Investigation, and the past president of the American Academy of

Hospice and Palliative Medicine. Dr. Abernethy received her M.D. at Duke University, where she also did her internal medicine residency, served as the chief resident, and completed her hematology/oncology fellowship. She received her Ph.D. from Flinders University in Australia, with a focus on evidence-based medicine and clinical informatics, and her bachelor's degree from the University of Pennsylvania.

John Balchunas, M.S., is the workforce director for The National Institute for Innovation in Manufacturing Biopharmaceuticals. In addition, Mr. Balchunas is responsible for business development and industry partnership for the professional development program at North Carolina State University's (NCSU's) Biomanufacturing Training and Education Center. Prior to joining NCSU in 2014, Mr. Balchunas served as the director of workforce development for the North Carolina Biotechnology Center (NCBiotech). As part of NCBiotech's education and training program for nearly 10 years, Mr. Balchunas forged an array of partnerships with industry to understand and communicate biopharmaceutical manufacturing workforce needs. Mr. Balchunas started his career as a technical writer in the biomanufacturing and medical diagnostic industries. He holds an M.S. in technical communication and a B.S. in microbiology from NCSU and was selected as a Marano Fellow in The Aspen Institute's 2012–2013 Sector Skills Academy.

William Bialek, Ph.D., received his A.B. and Ph.D. (1983) from the University of California, Berkeley. After postdoctoral stays in the Netherlands and the Institute for Theoretical Physics at the University of California, Santa Barbara, he returned to Berkeley to join the faculty in physics and biophysics (1986). At the end of 1990 he moved to the newly formed NEC Research Institute and then, in 2001, to Princeton University. Since 2009 he has also been a visiting faculty member at the Graduate Center of the City University of New York. Dr. Bialek is interested very broadly in whether it is possible to find theoretical principles that have the power and generality that people have come to expect in physics yet encompass the complexity and diversity of life's most beautiful phenomena. This search has led him to think about biological systems on many scales, including the dynamics of single-protein molecules, genetic networks in a developing embryo, neural coding and computation in the brain, and the collective behavior of animal groups. He is as passionate about teaching as about research, and he has had the pleasure of working with a stream of extraordinary young colleagues.

Adrian Bot, M.D., Ph.D., is the vice president and the global head of translational medicine at Kite, a Gilead Company, developing genetically engineered cell products for oncology indications. Dr. Bot has more than 20 years of experience in the biopharmaceutical industry with a focus on the discovery and development of immunotherapies. He obtained his M.D. in Romania in 1993 and his Ph.D. in biomedical sciences at the Mount Sinai School of Medicine in New York in 1998. Subsequently, he was a guest scientist at the Scripps Research Institute in La Jolla, California. Prior to his appointment as the chief scientific officer at Kite Pharma in 2011 and then the vice president of translational medicine, where he contributed to the development of first-in-class and breakthrough cell therapy products for cancer, Dr. Bot served in various senior research and development leadership positions at MannKind Corp and Alliance Pharmaceutical Corp in La Jolla, California. His prior and current activities and appointments include editorial boards (*Journal of Immunology*, *International Reviews of Immunology*), leadership appointments in global professional societies (Society for Immunotherapy of Cancer), and advisory boards (Elicio Therapeutics).

Atul Butte, M.D., Ph.D., is the Priscilla Chan and Mark Zuckerberg Distinguished Professor and the inaugural director of the Bakar Computational Health Sciences Institute at the University of California, San Francisco. Dr. Butte is also the chief data scientist for the entire University of California Health system, with 20 health professional schools, 6 medical schools, 5 academic medical centers, 10 hospitals, and more than 1,000 care delivery sites. Dr. Butte has been continually funded by the National Institutes of Health for 20 years, is an inventor on 24 patents, and has authored more than 200 publications, with research repeatedly featured in *The New York Times*, *The Wall Street Journal*, and *Wired* magazine. Dr. Butte was elected into the National Academy of Medicine in 2015, and in 2013 he was recognized by the Obama administration as a White House Champion of Change in Open Science for promoting science through publicly available data. Dr. Butte is also a founder of three investor-backed, data-driven companies: Personalis (initial public offering, 2019), which provides medical genome sequencing services; Carmenta (acquired by Progenity, 2015), which discovers diagnostics for pregnancy complications; and NuMedii, which finds new uses for drugs through open molecular data. Dr. Butte trained in computer science at Brown University, worked as a software engineer at Apple and Microsoft, received his M.D. at Brown University, trained in pediatrics and pediatric endocrinology at Children's Hospital Boston, then received his Ph.D. from the Harvard Medical School and the Massachusetts Institute of Technology.

Elana Fertig, Ph.D., runs a National Cancer Institute (NCI)-funded hybrid computational and experimental laboratory in the systems biology of cancer and therapeutic response. Her wet laboratory develops time-course models of therapeutic resistance and develops single-cell technologies. Her computational methods blend mathematical modeling and artificial intelligence to determine the biomarkers and molecular mechanisms of therapeutic resistance from multi-platform genomics data. These techniques have broad applicability beyond her resistance models, including notably to the analysis of clinical biospecimens, developmental biology, and neuroscience. Dr. Fertig is an associate professor of oncology and the assistant director of the Research Program in Quantitative Sciences and the associate director of the Convergence Institute at the Johns Hopkins University Sidney Kimmel Comprehensive Cancer Center, with secondary appointments in biomedical engineering and applied mathematics and statistics, affiliations in the Institute of Computational Medicine, the Center for Computational Genomics, machine learning, the Mathematical Institute for Data Science, and the Center for Computational Biology. Prior to entering the field of computational cancer biology, Dr. Fertig was a NASA research fellow in numerical weather prediction. Dr. Fertig's research is featured in more than 80 peer-reviewed publications, R/Bioconductor packages, and competitive funding portfolio as the principal investigator and the co-investigator. She serves on the editorial boards of the pre-eminent computational biology journals *PLOS Computational Biology* and *Cell Systems* and as a study section member for the NCI systems biology and informatics technology for cancer research study sections. Notably, she led the team that won the HPN-DREAM8 algorithm to predict phospho-proteomic trajectories from therapeutic response in cancer cells.

Paul Francois, Ph.D., is an associate professor in the Department of Physics at McGill University. His research focuses on the development of approaches inspired by statistical and computational physics for the theoretical understanding of the dynamics of biological systems and of their evolution. He works in close collaboration with experimentalists of a variety of systems, from embryonic development to early immune recognition.

Alison Gammie, Ph.D., is the director of the Division of Training, Workforce Development, and Diversity, which supports research training, career development, and diversity-building activities at the National Institute of General Medical Sciences (NIGMS). Prior to coming to NIGMS, she was a senior lecturer at Princeton University, where, in addition to teaching, mentoring, and running a research laboratory, she served as an academic advisor, an associate member at the Cancer Institute of New Jersey, and the director of diversity programs and graduate recruiting. Honors include Princeton's President's Award for Distinguished Teaching, the Graduate Mentoring Award, and the American Society for Microbiology Hinton Award for advancing the research careers of underrepresented minorities.

Sui Huang, M.D., Ph.D., is a molecular and cell biologist with a strong background in theoretical biology. He has devoted his research to understanding the very phenomenon of cancer from a complex systems perspective. Life scientists now readily acknowledge that the "whole is more than the sum of its parts," but the question is: What exactly is the "more" that we need in order to understand the "whole"? Can this abstract philosophical notion be reduced to a rigorous formal concept and concrete molecular entities? Pursuing this question has guided Dr. Huang's research in cancer and cell biology over the past decade. Before joining the Institute for Systems Biology (ISB) in fall 2011, Dr. Huang held faculty positions at the University of Calgary (Institute of Biocomplexity and Informatics), where he helped establish biocomplexity as a discipline in research and teaching, and at the Harvard Medical School (Children's Hospital), where he obtained the first experimental evidence for the existence of high-dimensional attractors in mammalian gene regulatory networks. Dr. Huang grew up in Geneva and Zurich. He received his M.D. from the University of Zurich and obtained thereafter, as the first recipient of the Ph.D.-Program-for-Physicians Award of the Swiss National Science Foundation, his Ph.D. in molecular biology and physical chemistry for work on interferons. As a postdoctoral fellow at Children's Hospital Boston, he investigated tumor angiogenesis and cell growth control. In that period, he also studied dynamical systems through his affiliation with the New England Complex Systems Institute. Seeing how both interferons and anti-angiogenic agents have failed to live up to their celebrated promise of curing cancer has had a lasting impact on Dr. Huang's views. The humbling recognition of the profound complexity of the living state fostered the desire to overcome the orthodoxy of reductionist, monocausal and deterministic thinking that prevailed in biomedicine and to put to use his knowledge of complex systems theory in his experimental research. Time was ripe in the late 1990s because the arrival of the "omics" technologies, and systems biology paved the way toward this interdisciplinary approach. With his move to ISB, Dr. Huang continues to unite experiment and theory to gain insights into the essence of multicellularity and cancer.

Iya Khalil, Ph.D., is the global head of the AI Innovation Center at Novartis. She is a technology entrepreneur and a physicist with a vision of transforming medicine and health care into a discipline that is quantitative, predictive, and patient-centric via artificial intelligence (AI) and big data. Prior to coming to Novartis, Dr. Khalil co-founded two AI and machine learning companies, Gene Network Sciences Inc. and GNS Healthcare, and was the co-inventor of the proprietary AI and machine learning software platform that underpins both entities. Dr. Khalil's machine learning and AI expertise spans 18 years with applications in drug discovery, drug development, clinical trial optimization, real-world evidence and pharmaceutical commercial applications, and all the way to treatment algorithms that can be applied at the point of care. She is a frequent speaker at industry conferences including Exponential Medicine, Milken Global Conference, Health 2.0, SXSW, Bio, and TEDx and was recently profiled in *Forbes* magazine as one of the women making AI more accessible and less scary. Dr. Khalil has published extensively in AI and machine learning for health care, including peer-reviewed journal articles and poster presentations at scientific conferences. She was recognized by President Obama in 2014 as a leading entrepreneur in genomic medicine and more recently named to *Inc.* magazine's list of top female founders of 2018. Dr. Khalil received her Ph.D. and M.S. in physics from Cornell University. Dr. Khalil is also fluent in Arabic. She is also a passionate member of Springboard enterprises, the largest network of innovators, investors, and influencers who are dedicated to building high-growth women-led technology companies.

Theresa Kotanchek, Ph.D., is the chief executive officer of Evolved Analytics LLC, a data science and analytics system and software provider (www.evolved-analytics.com). Using proprietary algorithms, evolved analytics discovers elusive relationships in complex data systems, extracting new insights and knowledge. Evolved Analytics's suite of global solutions is broad, reaching across multiple industry sectors, enabling new catalyst, drug, and materials discoveries; enhanced business forecasting; supply chain planning and logistics; and automated process and quality control. Prior to assuming her current role, Dr. Kotanchek spent 23 years in executive and leadership positions at Dow Chemical, including the vice president for sustainable technologies, innovation sourcing, and information research; the chief technology officer of Dow Chemical China Company Limited; the global business director of Dow Ventures; the global research and development director of Dow Plastics; and the corporate director of materials science and engineering. Dr. Kotanchek holds a doctorate in materials science and engineering, a master of science in ceramic science, and a bachelor of science in ceramic science and engineering from The Pennsylvania State University. She is currently the vice chair of the National Academies of Sciences, Engineering, and Medicine's National Materials and Manufacturing Board and has served as a member of the Committee on Foundational Best Practices for Making Value in America. Internationally recognized, she has given more than 200 invited lectures, published more than 100 technical articles, and holds 6 U.S. patents.

Jane Lebkowski, Ph.D., has been actively involved in the development of cell and gene therapies since 1986 and is the president of research and development (R&D) at Regenerative Patch Technologies (RPT), a biotechnology firm developing composite stem cell–based implants to restore retinal architecture and function in patients with macular degeneration. In this role Dr. Lebkowski oversees all of RPT's operations. From 2013 to 2017, Dr. Lebkowski also served as the chief scientific officer and the president of R&D at Asterias Biotherapeutics Inc., where she headed all preclinical, product, regulatory, and clinical development of Asterias's regenerative medicine and dendritic cell based–cancer immunotherapy products. Prior to joining Asterias, Dr. Lebkowski was the senior vice president of regenerative medicine and the chief scientific officer at Geron Corporation. Dr. Lebkowski led Geron's human embryonic stem cell program from 1998–2012 and was responsible for all research, preclinical development, product development, manufacturing, and clinical development activities supporting cell-based therapies for several regenerative medicine indications including spinal cord injury and cardiovascular disease. From 1986–1998, Dr. Lebkowski was the vice president of R&D at Applied Immune Sciences, where she directed activities to develop T cell–based cancer immunotherapies for solid tumors, hematologic malignancies, and AIDS. Following the acquisition of Applied Immune Sciences by Rhone Poulenc Rorer (RPR, currently Sanofi), Dr. Lebkowski remained at RPR as the vice president of discovery research. During Dr. Lebkowski's tenure at RPR, she coordinated preclinical investigations of gene therapy approaches for the treatment of cancer, cardiovascular disease, and nervous system disorders and directed vector formulations and delivery development. Dr. Lebkowski received her Ph.D. in biochemistry from Princeton University in 1982 and completed a postdoctoral fellowship at the Department of Genetics at Stanford University in 1986. Dr. Lebkowski has published more than 80 peer-reviewed publications and has 13 issued U.S. patents. Dr. Lebkowski has served on the board of directors of the American Society of Gene & Cell Therapy (ASGCT) and on numerous scientific advisory boards and professional committees including those supported by ASGCT and International Society for Stem Cell Research.

Bala Manian, Ph.D., has been a part of the Silicon Valley entrepreneurial community over the past four decades as an entrepreneur, an investor, and an innovator. Dr. Manian has been a founder or a co-founder of a large number of successful life sciences and medical technology companies in Silicon Valley over that 40 years. Before the Silicon Valley experience, he was an academic, as a member of the teaching faculty at the University of Rochester. An expert in the design of electro-optical systems, Dr. Manian is a prime driver behind many successful commercial products. While his educational training is in physics and engineering, his contributions have centered predominantly in life sciences and medical technology. As example of cross-disciplinary convergence, in February 1999 the Academy of Motion Picture Arts and Sciences awarded Dr. Manian a technical Academy Award for advances in digital cinematography. He has been recognized through several awards for his contributions as an educator, an inventor, and an entrepreneur. Dr. Manian holds more than 50 patents, many of which have resulted in successful commercial products. Dr. Manian received a B.S. in physics from Loyola College in Chennai, a postgraduate level diploma in instrumentation from the Madras Institute of Technology in Chennai, an M.S. in applied optics from the University of Rochester, and a Ph.D. in mechanical engineering from Purdue University.

Douglas Olson, Ph.D., received his bachelor's degree in chemistry from Maryville College and his Ph.D. in medicinal chemistry from Purdue University. Most of Dr. Olson's career has been spent in the medical device and in vitro diagnostics industry. He served as the president of Diagnostic Products Corporation's instrument systems division and as the corporate chief scientific officer prior to its sale to Siemens Health Care. Dr. Olson is the holder of eight U.S. patents and the author of a number of publications. He is a cancer survivor and patient number two in the initial University of Pennsylvania chimeric antigen receptor T cell clinical trial. He is a former member of the board of directors of the Eastern Pennsylvania chapter of the Leukemia & Lymphoma Society and is on the board of directors of Bühlmann Laboratories and Bühlmann Diagnostics Corp and currently serves as the president and the chief executive officer of Bühlmann Diagnostics Corp.

Larsson Omberg, Ph.D., M.Sc., is the vice president of systems biology at Sage Bionetworks and oversees a research agenda that focuses on both genomics and participant-centered research where data are being collected using remote sensors and mobile phones. The group focuses heavily on using open and team-based science to get a large number of external partners to collaborate on data-intensive problems. Dr. Omberg has a background in computational biology and has been developing computational methods for genomics analysis and disease modeling. Dr. Omberg obtained an M.Sc. in engineering physics from the Royal Institute of Technology in Stockholm, Sweden, and a Ph.D. from The University of Texas at Austin in physics before performing a postdoctoral fellowship in computational biology and biostatistics at Cornell University.

Anne Richelle, Ph.D., completed her Ph.D. in the Engineering Department of Université Libre de Bruxelles on the modeling, optimization, and control of yeast fermentation processes. After a first postdoc at the same university focused on the metabolic modeling of mammalian cells, she joined the lab of N. E. Lewis at the University of California, San Diego, to work on the integrated modeling of genotype–phenotype relationship in Chinese hamster ovary (CHO) cells, research for which she received the Eli Lilly Innovation

Fellowship Award. She is currently working at GlaxoSmithKline on the integration of systems biology tools from a process engineering perspective.

Sally Temple, Ph.D., is the scientific director of the Neural Stem Cell Institute (NSCI) and oversees scientific programs with the goal of understanding the role of neural stem cells in central nervous system development, maintenance, and repair. A native of York, England, Dr. Temple leads a team of 30 researchers focused on using neural stem cells to develop therapies for eye, brain, and spinal cord disorders. In 2008 she was awarded the MacArthur Fellowship Award for her contribution and future potential in the neural stem cell field. Dr. Temple received her undergraduate degree from Cambridge University, Cambridge, United Kingdom, specializing in developmental biology and neuroscience. She performed her Ph.D. work in optic nerve development at University College London, United Kingdom. She received a Royal Society fellowship to support her postdoctoral work at Columbia University in New York where she focused on spinal cord development. In 1989 Dr. Temple discovered that the embryonic mammalian brain contained a rare stem cell that could be activated to proliferate in vitro and produce both neurons and glia. Since then, her laboratory has continued to make pioneering contributions to the field of stem cell research by characterizing neural stem cells and the intrinsic and environmental factors that regulate their behavior. Her laboratory's research on the characterization of neural stem and progenitors brings us closer to developing effective clinical treatments for central nervous system damage in which tissue is lost, for example, due to neurodegenerative diseases or trauma. As the scientific director of NSCI, Dr. Temple oversees the research mission from basic to translational projects. Dr. Temple is a member of the board of directors and is a past president of the International Society for Stem Cell Research.

Dawn Tilbury, Ph.D., leads the Directorate for Engineering at the National Science Foundation (NSF) in its mission to support engineering research and education critical to the nation's future and to foster innovations to benefit society. Engineering breakthroughs address national challenges, such as smart manufacturing, resilient infrastructure, and sustainable energy systems. Engineering also brings about new opportunities in areas ranging from advanced photonics to prosthetic devices. The Engineering Directorate helps to advance NSF's Ten Big Ideas, including the Future of Work at the Human-Technology Frontier, the Quantum Leap, Understanding the Rules of Life, and NSF INCLUDES. The Engineering Directorate provides about 40 percent of the federal funding for fundamental research in engineering at academic institutions and distributes about 1,600 research awards each year. Partnerships with industry are a key component of the

Engineering Directorate's programs, including GOALI (Grant Opportunity for Academic Liaison with Industry) where industry researchers collaborate directly on academic research projects, and INTERN, which allows graduate students funded on NSF projects to spend up to 6 months in a non-academic internship (such as a company, government laboratory, or nonprofit organization). The Industry-University Cooperative Research Center program brings together NSF researchers with funding provided by industry and other government agencies to do pre-competitive research, and the ERC (Engineering Research Center) program supports large-scale convergence research projects together with workforce development, diversity and inclusion, and an innovation ecosystem. The Engineering Directorate coordinates NSF's I-Corps program, providing entrepreneurial training to faculty, graduate students, and postdocs. NSF's Small Business Innovation Research and Small Business Technology Transfer programs, housed in the Engineering Directorate, support fundamental research being done in high-tech small businesses helping them transition new technologies into the commercial marketplace. A professor at the University of Michigan since 1995, in both mechanical and electrical engineering, Dr. Tilbury has a background in systems and control engineering. She received a B.S. in electrical engineering, summa cum laude, from the University of Minnesota in 1989, and an M.S. and a Ph.D. in electrical engineering and computer sciences from the University of California, Berkeley, in 1992 and 1994, respectively. She is the inaugural chair of the Robotics Steering Committee and served as an associate dean for research in the College of Engineering. She was elected a fellow of the Institute of Electrical and Electronics Engineers in 2008 and a fellow of the American Society of Mechanical Engineers in 2012, and she is a life member of the Society of Women Engineers. Dr. Tilbury retains her position with the University of Michigan and shall return after her term with NSF expires.

Seshu Tyagarajan, Ph.D., is the global head of late-stage chemistry, manufacturing, and control (CMC) strategy for Novartis cell and gene therapy (CGT) and technical operations (NTO). She has 20 years of experience in the biopharmaceutical industry at companies such as Merck, Roche, Phyton, Biogen, and Eli Lilly. She holds an M.S. in bioengineering from Purdue University and a Ph.D. in chemical engineering from Rutgers University. Dr. Tyagarajan's career has spanned biologics and the cell and gene therapy space in the areas of CMC team leadership, current good manufacturing processes manufacturing, manufacturing sciences, and research and development. Her current responsibilities include successful transition of CGT pivotal trials into the manufacturing organization (NTO) and overseeing artificial intelligence collaborations for the cell and gene space.

Ben Wang, Ph.D., holds the Gwaltney Chair in Manufacturing Systems and is a professor in the Stewart School of Industrial and Systems Engineering, and a professor in the School of Materials Science and Engineering at the Georgia Institute of Technology. In addition, he serves as the executive director of the Georgia Tech Manufacturing Institute. Dr. Wang is a fellow of the Institute of Industrial Engineers, the Society of Manufacturing Engineers, and the Society for the Advancement of Material and Process Engineering. From 2017 to 2019 he served as the chair of the National Materials and Manufacturing Board at the National Academies of Sciences, Engineering, and Medicine. In those 3 years the board oversaw several landmark studies, including A Vision for Center-Based Engineering Research, A Quadrennial Review of the National Nanotechnology Initiative, Frontiers of Materials Research: A Decadal Survey, and Strategic Long-Term Participation by DOD in Its Manufacturing USA Institutes. Dr. Wang's professional focus is on strengthening manufacturing competitiveness through technology, infrastructure, workforce, and policy. In addition to authoring or co-authoring more than 260 refereed journal papers, he is a co-author of 3 books and has a portfolio of issued and applied-for patents that now exceeds 35, 15 of which have been licensed or are in discussion for commercialization. Dr. Wang earned his bachelor's degree in industrial engineering from Tunghai University (Taiwan) and his master's degree and Ph.D. in industrial engineering from The Pennsylvania State University.

Robert Zambon, Ph.D., is the Real-World Innovation Leader in Janssen Scientific Affairs at Janssen Pharmaceuticals. In his role, Dr. Zambon leads and supports strategic innovation initiatives for Janssen Scientific Affairs focused on the usage of innovative technologies, analytics, data, and partnerships to accelerate and advance real-world research and initiatives across all of Janssen's therapeutic areas. Dr. Zambon has close to 20 years of experience in the life sciences industry with experience in strategy development, program management, clinical research, product development, sales force training, client management, regulatory affairs, analytics, and market research. He has led and supported research programs in the areas of cardiology, orthopedics, immunology, infectious disease, and medical countermeasures. Dr. Zambon received his Ph.D. in molecular and cell biology at the University of Maryland and his B.S. in biotechnology at Rutgers University.

Peter Zandstra, Ph.D., graduated with a bachelor of engineering degree from McGill University in the Department of Chemical Engineering, obtained his Ph.D. from The University of British Columbia (UBC) in the Department of Chemical Engineering and Biotechnology, and continued his research training as a postdoctoral fellow in the field of bioengineering at the Massachusetts Institute of Technology. Dr. Zandstra is the chief scientific officer for CCRM, the founding director of the School of Biomedical Engineering at UBC, and the director of the Michael Smith Laboratories at UBC. He holds an academic appointment as a professor at the University of Toronto's Institute of Biomaterials and Biomedical Engineering. He is the Canada Research Chair in Stem Cell Bioengineering and is a recipient of a number of awards and fellowships including the Premiers Research Excellence Award (2002), the E.W.R. Steacie Memorial Fellowship (2006), the John Simon Guggenheim Memorial Foundation Fellowship (2007), Canada's Top 40 Under 40 (2008), the University of Toronto's McLean Award (2009), and the Till and McCulloch Award (2013). Dr. Zandstra is also a fellow of the American Institute for Medical and Biological Engineering, the American Association for the Advancement of Science, and the Royal Society of Canada. His research focuses on understanding how complex communication networks between stem cells and their progeny influence self-renewal and differentiation and how this information can be applied to the design of novel culture technologies capable of controlling cell fate.

Appendix C

Statement of Task

The current approach to characterizing the quality of a regenerative medicine product and the manufacturing process often involves measuring as many endpoints as possible, but this approach has proved to be inadequate and unsustainable. To explore how cross-disciplinary systems thinking approaches can support the identification of relevant quality attributes and streamline manufacturing and regulatory processes of regenerative medicine products, a planning committee of the National Academies of Sciences, Engineering, and Medicine will hold a public workshop. Speakers at the workshop may be asked to discuss new advances in data acquisition, data analysis, and theoretical frameworks and how systems approaches can be applied to the development of regenerative medicine products that can address the unmet needs of patients. Discussions may explore how systems thinking is currently being applied in clinical and manufacturing settings. The planning committee will develop the workshop agenda, select and invite speakers and discussants, and may moderate the discussions. A proceedings of the workshop will be prepared by a designated rapporteur in accordance with institutional guidelines.